The International Library

CONSTITUTION-TYPES IN DELINQUENCY

ARBOR SCIENTIÆ
ARBOR VITÆ

Founded by C. K. Ogden

The International Library of Psychology

ABNORMAL AND CLINICAL PSYCHOLOGY
In 19 Volumes

CONSTITUTION-TYPES IN DELINQUENCY

Practical Applications and Bio-Physiological Foundations of Kretschmer's Types

W A WILLEMSE

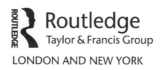

Routledge
Taylor & Francis Group

LONDON AND NEW YORK

First published in 1932 by
Routledge, Trench, Trubner & Co., Ltd.
2 Park Square, Milton Park, Abingdon, Oxfordshire OX14 4RN
711 Third Avenue, New York, NY 10017

First issued in paperback 2014

Routledge is an imprint of the Taylor and Francis Group, an informa business

© 1932 W A Willemse

British Library Cataloguing in Publication Data
A CIP catalogue record for this book
is available from the British Library

Constitution-Types in Delinquency
ISBN 0415-20937-4
Abnormal and Clinical Psychology: 19 Volumes
ISBN 0415-21123-9
The International Library of Psychology: 204 Volumes
ISBN 0415-19132-7

ISBN 13: 978-1-138-88240-9 (pbk)
ISBN 13: 978-0-415-20937-3 (hbk)

CONTENTS

v

PREFACE

THIS work has two main aims :—

First : To apply the clinically originated constitution-psychological typology of Kretschmer (with the extensions of Delbrück, Pfahler, etc.) to male juvenile delinquents. This typology roots in the mental clinic, but is of application to all fundamental manifestations of personality differences : scientists, artists, rulers, but also delinquents. It is a special task to work out its applications to each of these fields of manifestation. Our task has been to establish, preliminarily, how the various qualities such as autism, perseveration, sociable integration with the environment, insensitivity, drivenness, etc., are manifested in all the mental dispositions and functions connected with crime. In this way our work touched here and there on general problems, such as heredity, emotional disturbances, etc., already treated exhaustively by other investigators. But it always remains an approach under a more specialized view-point —the bio-typological or constitution-typological one. As such it can in no way, and does not aspire to, replace or refute the classical works of Burt, Healy, and others on juvenile delinquents.

Secondly : To co-ordinate—as far as it was possible within the specialized framework—the bio-typologies of Kretschmer, Jaensch, Pende, Berman, Wiersma, etc., in so far as there appears to be similarity between the underlying biological principles of these typologies and those of Kretschmer's typology. For this purpose I have tried to discuss the bio-physiological bases of the types as fundamentally as the present development of science permits. These discussions and expositions may perhaps also serve to direct the attention of English and American investigators to the interesting bio-typological studies, now being made at different centres on the Continent.

This work is one of the products of investigations made by our Institute on vocational, industrial, and social adjustment of juveniles. The Union Department of

vii

Education supported these investigations financially and morally, and it is our pleasure to express here our sincere appreciation of that support. We have to thank the Union Director of Prisons, as well, for kind permission to work at Reformatories, and also the wardens and teachers of reformatories and industrial schools for valuable assistance.

In a more personal strain I have to state that I owe much gratitude to Dr. P. Skawran, the Director of our Institute at Pretoria. He urged me to the experimental-psycho-pathological approach of psychology on the lines of Störring (Bonn), of whom he is a deserving student. The psychological works of Störring, in their emphasis on the feeling and volitional side of the mind, particularly as analysed with the aid of psychopathological material, have been, since Skawran's sound introduction of them to me, the basis of my studies.

I am furthermore much indebted to Professor T. Hugo. He introduced me to the psychical monism of Heymans and of Paulsen, which has provided me with a firm philosophical basis and justification for these studies on the relations between body and mind.

In this way I was absorbed by the continental investigations which I shall endeavour to bring to the notice of my countrymen in this work. Community of scientific interest is, to my mind, a potent factor in the establishment of true internationality.

W. A. WILLEMSE.

PSYCHOLOGICAL LABORATORY,
UNIVERSITY OF PRETORIA.

April, 1931.

CHAPTER I

PROBLEMS AND AIMS

1. *The Relation between the Delinquent Act and the Personality*

During the last fifty years the attitude towards crime has changed fundamentally. Where formerly the act of crime and its immediate external causes were placed in the centre of importance, the modern schools of penal justice attach more importance to the criminal himself—to his personality. " The convict's attitude towards justice, his entire past, and what is to be expected from him in the future must determine the nature and duration of his punishment," said the well-known authority v. Liszt [1] at the beginning of this century when he opposed the views of the classical school. Particularly, the punishment was no longer inflicted as a rehabilitation of the violated sense of justice of the community. Punishment had gradually come to be a measure either to reform the delinquent, or, if he were irreclaimable, to protect society from his onslaughts. Moreover, it is not only on the disposition to crime of a particular nature that more stress is now laid, but the Austrian School of Criminal Biology under Lenz,[2] and the Bavarian grading system of punishment (Stufenstrafvollzug) particularly,[3] have in the last decade extended the field of investigation and consideration from the criminal dispositions to the entire bio-psychological personality. The criminal act, accordingly, appears as the realization (Aktualisiering)

---

[1] *Strafrechtliche Aufsätze und Vorträge*, Bd. 2, p. 57.
[2] A. Lenz, *Grundriss der Kriminalbiologie*.
[3] *Der Stufenstrafvollzug*, published in 3 volumes by the Bavarian Ministry of Justice. These works must be referred to for detailed treatment. I shall only touch these magnificent systems in so far .as they relate to my special theme.

of a potential functional system, and this system includes mental as well as bio-physiological factors. All these part-functions must be understood or explained in their interrelations in an organic, unitary and structural whole of the psychophysical individuality.[1]

The American psychiatrist Healy,[2] and the British psychologist Cyril Burt,[3] have (mainly since 1910) made similar studies on all the factors causally connected with delinquency in Juveniles. The intelligence, emotional and volitional peculiarities, and also physical qualities of a very large material have been carefully considered by these authors. But their approach of the individual delinquent in his mental and physical make-up is not identical to that of the German-Austrian biological school. Some of their findings, such as infantilisms, physical over-development, etc., have a very intimate connection with our bio-types. The main aim of Healy and Burt, however, was general causal relationships, rather than typological studies. The bio-typological approach of the delinquent, as compared with these very valuable yet general treatments, will become clear as we proceed.

The study of the delinquent personality, therefore—both typologically and generally—has in our time become so self-evident that we are inclined to look down upon the earlier attitude with some vexation. We know now that punishment is not the only problem that demands a profound study of the psycho-biological personality; Professor Mezger shows very lucidly that all three of the main problems of criminal procedure—(a) Imputability (responsibility), (b) Corrigibility, and (c) Punishment, can only be solved when the adequacy (correspondence, agreement) of the act of crime to the full personality, and the adequacy of the personality to his environment is obvious. Discrepancies between personality and act, and discrepancies between personality and environment, call for further investigation before any of the three

[1] A. Lenz, "Mitteilungen der Kriminal biologischen Gesellschaft," *Dresden Tagung*, 1928, p. 123.
[2] Healy, *The Individual Delinquent*, Boston, 1924.
[3] Burt, *The Young Delinquent*, London, 1927.

problems can be attacked.[1] It must, however, from the outset be distinctly understood that with this emphasis on the entire bio-psychological personality no support is given to the theory that the delinquent personality is a distinct species or atavistic degeneration as proposed by Lombroso. This writer deserves much admiration for what he has done to direct attention on the whole personality of the criminal and strongly also on the bio-physiological concomitants of severe criminality. But criminality is not a biological or psychological unity connected with a definite unitary type.[2] Grühle tries to make this clearer by stating that criminality is a form of life (Lebensform) and not a type.[3] From the social and ethical points of view the various criminal manifestations seem to have more in common than when they are considered from a psychological or biological point of view. The same confusion between social and normic (teleological) types on the one hand with bio-psychological (etiological) types on the other hand, is also made in other fields, e.g. psychopathy, where the " unstable " (Haltlosen) are more of a social economic (teleological) class than a bio-psychological (etiological) type, because the bio-psychological causes (etiology) of instability may be very different in different members of this class.[4] The extreme diversity and complexity of types of criminal personalities will become more and more obvious as progress is made in the study of psycho-biological types and their biological types, and their application to criminalities.

2. Intelligence of Delinquents

When more emphasis came to be laid on the delinquent himself, instead of on the delinquent act, the first tendency

---

[1] *Mitteilungen der Kr. Bio. Ges.*, pp. 32, 96.

[2] Hapke, *Zeitschrift f. Angewandte Psycho.*, Bd. 33, p. 13, and Kretschmer *Physique and Character*, London, 1925.

[3] *Mitteilungen*, p. 19.

[4] *Vide* K. Schneider, *Die Psychopathischen Persönlichkeiten*, Leipzig, 1928, p. 29.

was to attach most importance to a cognitive aspect of the personality—his intelligence. Goddard (1914), the authority on feeble-mindedness, is very sweeping in his emphasis on mental deficiency as the main cause of crime. He points out that the attitude towards the delinquent has gone through an evolution. It has developed from the old idea of vengeance by the god, Justice, to the principle of punishment as a deterrent, and, finally, to the more recent one of understanding him, of treatment and reformation. But studies on the environment, according to Goddard, have shown that there is a limit beyond which the congenital endowment does not allow its possessor to improve. There is a limit of responsibility, too. Feeble-mindedness explains the criminal type better than does hereditary criminality. " The so-called criminal type is merely a type of feeble-mindedness, a type misunderstood and mistreated, driven into criminality for which he is well fitted by nature." [1] He goes on to give the percentages of feeble-mindedness from sixteen institutions for delinquents which show that " an estimate of 50 per cent is well within the limit ". But he admits that the higher controls are also defective, thus already indicating the importance of temperament and character factors. In fact, he mentions that the other factors apart from intelligence defects are : environment and temperament ; and in his special treatment of Delinquency, Goddard particularly states that " no greater contribution to the problem of delinquency has ever been made than the concept of the psychopathic child ".[2] The psychopathic child is, as we shall see, one who has an unbalanced temperament and character. It is significant also that Goddard found a comparatively small amount of crime in his family histories of feeble-mindedness (10 per cent). Another authority who investigated several hundreds of juveniles in the Chicago clinic, and published his monumental work in 1915,[3] viz. W. Healy, also strongly

---

[1] Goddard, *Feeble-mindedness, its cause and consequents*, New York, 1914, 1923, pp. 6–10.
[2] Goddard, *Juvenile Delinquency*, 1921, p. 28.
[3] Healy, *The Individual Delinquent*, Boston, 1914 and 1924, p. 447.

emphasized mental deficiency as a cause of crime. "Undoubtedly 10 to 30 per cent, or even more, of prison and reformatory population, if tested, would be shown to be feeble-minded"; and further "mental defect forms the largest single cause of delinquency".

Later investigations, however, have shown that though intelligence defects are significant, especially in juveniles, first offenders, and sex offenders, the emotional, impulse and volitional side of the delinquent personality deserves foremost importance. Cyril Burt's book is based on intimate knowledge of a large city; material and elaborate tests prove conclusively that the intelligence factor, though "notable", cannot explain the bulk of delinquent personalities: only 8 per cent of the children tested "are backward in intelligence by at least three-tenths of their ages".[1] Another significant feature of the intellectual life of delinquents clearly isolated by Burt is their backwardness in education attainments. This fact, fully corroborated by the later researches still to be mentioned, indicates either a detrimental environment or defects on the emotional and will side of delinquent personalities. Brooks (1929),[2] points out that juvenile delinquency is not so simple as would appear from early investigations on feeble-mindedness. He shows that 75 per cent of a group of 1,212 juvenile repeated offenders have I.Q.s above the 80 level (limit of mental deficiency) of the Stanford-Binet scale. He also quotes Healy and Bronner's later studies which show that in 4,000 juvenile repeated offenders 72·6 were "definitely mentally normal". A recent investigation by Slawson (1926),[3] led to the following conclusions in regard to the intelligence degree as a cause of Delinquency: (a) "In verbal abstract intelligence, largely indicative of scholastic success, the boys are very inferior to non-delinquent children." (b) This inferiority is less marked in non-verbal concrete intelligence. (c) Tested with the Stenquist Mechanical Aptitude Test,

[1] Cyril Burt, *The Young Delinquent*, London, 1925 and 1927, p. 300.
[2] Brooks, *Psychology of Adolescence*, New York, 1929, p. 405.
[3] Slawson, *The Delinquent Boy*, Boston, 1926, p. 191.

the delinquent boys were even slightly superior to a normal group. (*d*) The results of questionnaires on defective emotional make-up filled in by the boys show an intimate association between this and delinquency. Perhaps the most magnificent study in this direction is that by Professor Murchison.[1] He compared the results of the Army Alfa Test applied to the soldiers from various States with a large number of prisoners from the same States. The general conclusions reached by Professor Murchison in regard to our present problem are the following :—

(*a*) " In terms of Alpha scores the criminal group seems superior to the white draft group " (soldiers).
(*b*) " Crimes of deception and fraud are committed by men of no mean ability," " more than half are superior individuals." " About half the individuals who commit crimes against sex are inferior individuals."
(*c*) " Recidivists seem more intelligent than are first offenders," but not in all the types of crime. In fraud the first offenders being more intelligent.
(*d*) The criminal group is much less literate than the army.

Murchison accordingly admits that temperament may possibly play the chief rôle in the commission of all crime.

In this connection, the argument of Hapke [2] is also interesting. Hapke, working under Professor Stern of Hamburg, argues that real criminality plays a relatively insignificant rôle in the members of the famous feeble-minded families investigated : Criminality in the family Kallikak, 0·3%; Rufer, 1·0%; Nam, 1·0%; Pehr, 2·0%; Markus, 2·0%; Hill Folk, 4·0%; Dack, 4·0%; Juke, 6·0%; Zero, 7·0%; Viktoria, 39·0%; Anable, 88·0%. The high percentages in the last two cases Hapke explains as due to the inclusion of insignificant home troubles, insults, false alarms, etc., in the inventory of crimes.

Our own results tally to a large extent with the post-war researches. In arithmetical (Fig. 1), geometrical

---

[1] Carl Murchison, *Criminal Intelligence*, Massachusetts, 1926.
[2] *Zeitschrift f. Angewandte Psych.*, Bd. 33, p. 18.

(Fig. 4), and algebraical (Fig. 2) calculations, the reformatory boys of Tokai, with an average age of 16–19 years, perform more or less equally to the South African trade-school boy of a similar age. It is striking, however, that there is always a certain group among the delinquents

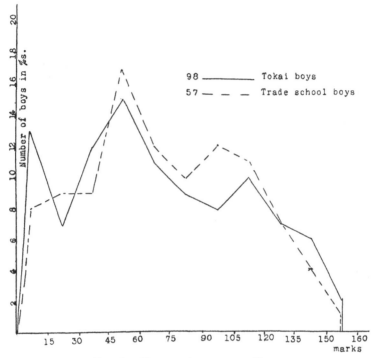

98 —————— Tokai boys

57 — _ — Trade school boys

Fig. 1.—Mental Arithmetic Test.

who are very inferior, even though the bulk coincides with the non-delinquents. This corresponds to a finding of most of the earlier investigators, including Murchison, and may to some extent explain the over-emphasis laid in pre-war works on the question of feeble-mindedness. It must also be mentioned that in South Africa feeble-minded delinquents are to some extent isolated immediately after conviction. In mechanical aptitude (our special psycho-technical test) the results are also very interesting

(Fig. 3). A large number are below average, but more Tokai boys than trade-school boys come above 72 per cent. This indicates that on the practical intelligence side a good number of delinquents are very superior. In fact, in

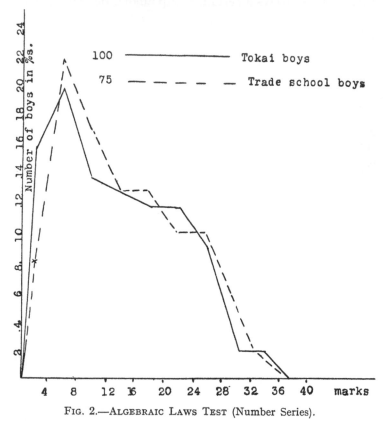

FIG. 2.—ALGEBRAIC LAWS TEST (Number Series).

a few cases, this exceptional endowment for practical concrete problems was a strong incentive to delinquency as the following example will illustrate :—

Case 1.—Age 17. Tests show that in logical sequence, complicated mental tasks and mathematics, he is brilliant if his interest is aroused. But his most outstanding abilities lie in originality, accuracy, and above all a remarkable insight into concrete mechanical problems. He is quick and energetic, but not at all reliable or persistent at monotonous routine occupation. Boyishly jovial, unreflective, undaunted, and self-willed. Just as fond of a good argument as an interesting mechanical problem.

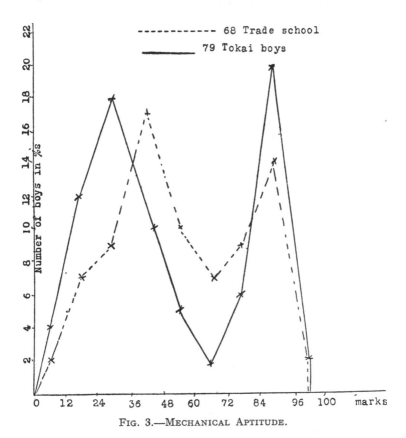

FIG. 3.—MECHANICAL APTITUDE.

Frequent change of work. About 15 charges against him (of which only four proved) for house-breaking and stealing. Entered stores and garages, etc., with special keys, or in such a way that the police were baffled in their efforts to discover his means of ingress. Stole cars for joy-rides out of garages and replaced them same night. Often took only a bunch of keys from a place to indicate that he had been inside. Spoils given to a relative. In interview it became completely evident that all his escapades were more of a Chinese puzzle and interesting problems which he both created and solved, than real criminal egotistic manifestations. He enjoys a housebreaking venture just as he enjoys an argument. For him, both are intellectual exercises which he likes to carry out successfully.

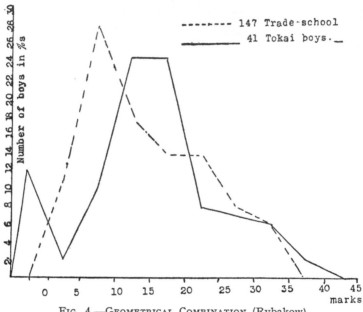

FIG. 4.—GEOMETRICAL COMBINATION (Rybakow).

Also, as far as manual skill is concerned, the results of Moede's ambidexterity test [1] show a complete correspondence between the Tokai reformatory boys and 114 trades-school boys tested all over the Union of S. Africa (Fig. 5). The educational attainments of the Tokai boys (100) show an average of Standard 5·2. This is certainly low when one considers that Standard 6, or the age of 16, is the compulsory limit set by the law for leaving school ; further, that the largest number come from towns where school education is within easy reach, and that most

[1] For particulars refer to F. Giese, *Handbuch Psycho-tech. Eignungsprüfungen*, Halle, 1925, p. 404.

skilled artizans have to reach the Standard 6 limit in order to be legally apprenticed. We must also bear in mind that all these boys are older than 17 years.

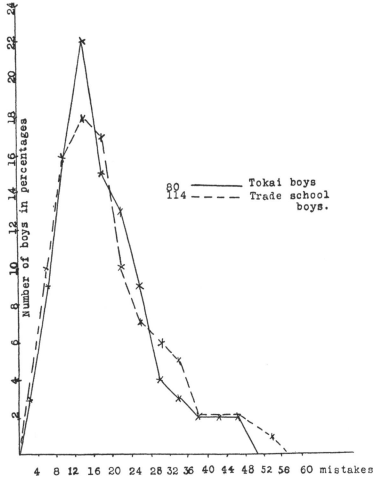

FIG. 5.—TWO-HAND TEST (cf. Moede).

Such a low standard of school attainment or literacy is, as Murchison has shown, more a symptom of other factors, such as temperament, tenacity, than of an inferior intelligence.

Our survey of previous investigations and own tests accordingly seem to justify the following conclusions :—

(a) The intelligence defect is not the main cause of delinquency.[1]

(b) Especially in juvenile delinquents a certain group appears to be remarkably weak in the more abstract intelligence.

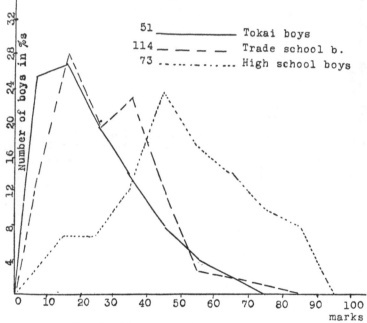

FIG. 6.—MEMORY FOR SENSEFUL MATERIAL.

(c) Juvenile delinquents appear to be generally weak in educational attainments.

(d) Temperamental and/or environmental factors must be all-important as causes of delinquency.

3.   *Temperament and Character factors in Delinquency*

Preliminarily, we may say that temperament and character comprise the emotional, impulse, and volitional factors in their widest applications.   We shall endeavour

[1] This view is also supported by the German-Austrian school of Criminology, *Stufenstrafvollzug*, 1929, p. 153.

to give more definite delineations in a later chapter. In the so-called psychopathic personalities, the abnormality pertains to temperament and character factors. Psychopathy is a functional disco-ordination, disproportion and unbalanced condition of the emotions, feelings, impulse-life, and activity.[1] It is difficult, though very necessary, to differentiate between psychopathy and real psychotic conditions. Jaspers and Schneider [2] proposed the criterium of comprehensibility, appreciability, possibility of empathy, in the case of psychopathy; whereas in the psychotic " process " the personality is transformed entirely and irreparably. The biological and physiological bases of the " process " are usually also inexplicable. Between the definitely insane and the entirely normal we find this wide characterological playground of psychopathy. The demarcations and definitions are very flowing and arbitrary. Bumke [3] says of them : " Fundamentally all these functional and psychopathic disturbances are rooted in the healthy mind and as soon as one investigates their first and most subtle manifestations they all finally dissolve into normal psychology." The race hygienist, F. Lenz, holds that psychopaths constitute 10 per cent of the general population.[4] This is also the opinion of Professors J. Lange and E. Rüdin from the Münich psychiatrical institute.[4] The criterium by which to distinguish them from real insanity is also fairly vague. Jaspers' suggestion, supported by Kurt Schneider, that " comprehensibility ", " appreciability ", " empathy ", is possible of the personalities of psychopaths, but not of the insane, is only partly valid : The researches of Bumke and Carl Schneider [5] on the real insanity of Schizophrenia, show that the mental life of these patients can within

[1] Birnbaum, *Psychopathische Verbrecher*, Leipzig, 1926, p. 10.
[2] Kurt Schneider, *Psychopathischen Persönlichkeiten*, Leipzig, 1928, p. 6.
[3] Bumke, *Die Grenzen der Geistige Gesundheit*, Munich, 1929.
[4] *Stufenstrafvollzug*, 1928 ; E. Rüdin, *Psychiatrische Indikation zur Sterilizierung*, 1928.
[5] Schneider, *Psychologie der Schizophrenen*, Leipzig, 1930. Much depends, of course, as van der Horst " Körperbau und Charakter", *Z'ischrift f. Neur. u. Psychiat*, Bd. 93, p. 421, has experimentally verified, on the temperament of the person who attempts to " understand ". Schizo-personalities understand Schizophrenes better.

limits also be "comprehended", "appreciated," viz. as a type of semi-sleep. However, we need not define the term "psychopath" closely. For our purpose it suffices to know that the term stands for temperamental and character abnormalities as distinguished from intelligence defects, and as such forms a very suitable field for the application of our typology. Since the "psychopaths" are not normal and also not insane, they present, as we shall see in our discussion of the psychopathological method, exactly the material for verification and further elaboration of the bio-typologies.

With regard to the rôle of psychopaths in criminality, many prominent authorities agree upon the wide prevalency of these people in delinquent material. Koch, one of the founders of the term, says : "I have never known a born criminal other than a psychopathic one."[1] Birnbaum states that in all criminal acts, psychopathic elements play the main part, and he mentions further on that v. Liszt, who still laid so much emphasis on the social (i.e. not personal) causes of crime, also took psychopathic strains as the most characteristic qualities of criminals. Throughout his classical treatment Birnbaum directs attention on the feeling factors as the main determinants in mental life, especially in motivation and action.[2] Similarly, Michel, of the school of legal medicine in Graz, Austria, in a very intensive investigation of 302 habitual criminals, found 249, i.e. 83 per cent to be psychopathic.[3] Reiss found 88 psychopaths in a total of 131 investigated severe criminals. Professor Kramer [4] found over a period of many years, at the juvenile court of Berlin, that 50 per cent of those convicted were mentally abnormal, and of these psychopaths formed a considerable part. Many other prominent authorities agree with this. In the relatives of delinquents, Professor Burt [5] (who prefers to

[1] Quoted by Michel, "Der Psychopath. Gew. Verbrecher" in *Mitteilungen der Krim. Bio*, 1928, p. 83.
[2] Birnbaum, *op. cit.*, p. 6, 19.
[3] *Mitteilungen*, 1928, p. 75.
[4] *Psychopath. Veranlagung und Straffälligkeit im Jugendalter*, Langenzalsa, 1920.
[5] Burt, *The Young Delinquent*, 1927, p. 52, 514, 422.

keep the term for a more advanced stage, qualitatively different from the normal, and therefore does not speak of psychopaths in this sense) found that " temperamental disturbances with moral symptoms not only recur far more frequently than any other one group—physical, intellectual, or psychopathological—they recur more frequently than the whole of the remainder put together." But also in the delinquents themselves Burt found that temperamental conditions (" instincts and emotions "), are of enormous importance as causes of crime.

On account of the flowing demarcations between border-line cases of temperamental and character disturbances and normal cases, we have in our own research not attempted a numerical determination of the psychopathy involved. On the psychical side we found numerous indubitable abnormalities such as strong distrust, inert, lame social response, explosive emotions, extremes of energy forms,[1] sexual perversions, extreme unreflective optimism, etc. In the sequel we shall have ample oppor-tunity to demonstrate such abnormal accentuation in the framework of our typology. The prevalence of these disturbances in our own material and in that of more experienced investigators seems to be unquestionable. This fact is a proof, too, of the importance of the feeling and volitional side of the mind in life as it has been emphasised in the works of Störring. But this fact also indicates the value of typological studies of temperament and character for the problems of delinquency ; on the other hand, in the light of our discussion on the value of the psychopathological method in studies on feelings and will, the wide prevalency of psychopaths in delinquent material promises a rich field to further our typology.

4. *Heredity and Delinquency*

We all begin to think biologically when we deal with life processes and it is, accordingly, not necessary to elaborate

[1] Skawran, " Typology of Ergograms," *Psycho-Tech. Ztschrift*, Berlin, 1931.

on the value of heredity or environment in the etiology of crime. For detailed, systematic treatments, the works of Burt and Healy must be consulted. We need only indicate the aspects relevant to our special form of approach. The psychopathic constitutions are generally accepted as hereditary or at any rate congenital.[1] As Bumke says, we cannot determine yet whether they are due to germ-injury, e.g. in alcoholic parents, or to hereditary germ structure. Psychopathy and crime, anyhow, are intimately connected according to our survey of the best informed investigations. Accordingly, much of the intrinsic criminal mind cannot be due to environment, but is congenitally determined. Also, the morphological features of an individual are generally taken to be relatively little influenced by the environment. Facial and body features are both popularly and scientifically taken to be largely hereditary.[2] If we are, therefore, able to indicate co-ordinations between delinquency and biophysiological constitutions, this will also indicate the importance of heredity. The studies in heredity by Mjöen, Hoffmann, Reiss, and Ziehen, however, give an entirely new face to the problem of the heredity of criminality. They show that a disposition to criminality or any other complex mental aptitude such as musical genius, leadership, etc., can be built up synthetically from hereditary factors in the different progenitors, which original factors by themselves may have been harmless in the case of delinquents, or worthless in the other two instances. Only the new biological synthesis produces the complex and strange result: an explosive father and an unstable mother = an outrageous thief.[3] Mjöen has in this way indicated

---

[1] Birnbaum, *Psychopatische Verbrecher*, 1926, p. 3.

[2] Dr. M. A. van Herwerden of the University of Utrecht in his book, *Erfelykheid by den Mensch en Eugenetiek*, 1926, p. 176. indicates that in many royal families (e.g. Bourbons, Habsburgs, Hohenzollern), a typical facial form or body-build could be clearly traced through many generations. Haecker, the geneticist, has shown the possible biological unity of various such feature complexes by reducing, for instance, the Habsburg typical face to functions of the pituitary gland.

[3] Hoffmann, *Das Problem des Character aufbaues*, etc., Berlin, 1926, p. 93, and Lange in *Stufenstraffvollsug*, 1928, p. 147. *Konstitution und Character*, edited by M. Hirsch, 1928.

that the literary genius Björnsterne Björnson inherited a plastic phantasy from one parental side and critical intellect from the other side. Only a happy combination of the two produced the genius.[1] Ziehen claims to have demonstrated that Schumann inherited musical taste from the maternal line and poetic phantasy from the paternal side.[1] If such inheritance-syntheses are possible, all psychopathy and similar disturbances in the ancestors of delinquents become exceedingly significant. Burt's finding of " intermittent outbursts of instinct and emotion " without being " flagrant breaches of the law ", and also his finding that of all environmental causes those centring about the family life are most disastrous,[2] become very significant under this new aspect. There is another similar aspect of inherited temperament which Hoffmann has shown to be very significant and that is antinomies, disharmonies, within the personality. Mutually antagonistic hereditary dispositions lead to temperamental and character disharmony and even to disruption of the personality in mental disease. It may, therefore, be possible that characteristics still normal in each of the parents will prove to be pathologically disharmonious when synthesized in the offspring, and so lead to un-expected manifestations.

The question of hereditary influences becomes more and more complicated with new discoveries in the field of human biology. Epilepsy, for instance, seems to depend, in so far as it is hereditary, on recessive factors, so that absence of the malady in the nearest progenitors does not exclude its heredity. The picture becomes more com-plicated when such recessive hereditary factors are at the same time sex-linked, or even more complicated when only transmittable in either the male or female gene-complex, as e.g. colour-blindness. Until all the problems of recessive factors, linkages, hereditary " unit characters ", have been better studied in human mental life, nothing can be decided. Even where there is definite environmental

---

[1] v. Herwerden, *op. cit.*, p. 270.
[2] Burt, *op. cit.*, pp. 56 and 187.

influence, as in trauma-epilepsy, the main cause may have been hereditary dispositions : Kreyenberg has proved in a material of 700 epileptics that trauma-epilepsy is also concomitant with definite somatic constitutional types.[1] Hoffmann formulates the relations between constitutional and environmental factors in these words : " All acquired qualities are only a new pronouncement (Ausprägung) of the constitution."[2] In some instances the constitution is the main determinant, in others the environment, but the constitution is always implicated. The researches of Lange[3] on identical and ordinary twins have shown that, as far as criminality is concerned, out of 13 pairs of identical twins 10 were strikingly concordant in their criminal dispositions, while out of 17 ordinary twins only 2 were concordant in their criminal dispositions. In the identical twins the time of first conviction and the nature of the crime were in many instances remarkably concordant without the twins having been subject to the same environment.   This seems to indicate that where the individuals developed on one and the same placenta, i.e. where the germ plasma and prenatal conditions were more or less identical, the subsequent careers proved to be strikingly concordant, but in individuals where the germ plasma and prenatal conditions (genes, different placenta, etc.) could be different, the subsequent careers proved to be discordant.   But though such experiments seem to indicate that the congenital determinants deserve pre-eminent consideration, we may readily admit that the environment acts pathoplastically on the delinquent outcome.   The environment provides the means through which the innate dispositions are manifested ; and especially in certain psychopathic cases the psychopathy consists in this extreme pliability, suggestibility and ease with which such individuals are misled.   Especially where psychopathy is complicated with feeble-mindedness— as is often the case according to Birnbaum—the environ-

[1] " Körperbau, Epilepsie, und Charakter," *Zeitschrift f. d. Ges. Neurologie und Psychiatrie*, Bd. 112, p. 506.
[2] Hoffmann, *op. cit.*, p. 166.
[3] *Verbrechen als Schicksal* (Criminality as Fate), Leipzig, 1929.

ment will have strong influence. Also, we do not really co-ordinate certain forms of bodily constitution with delinquency as a whole, as Lombroso attempted to do ; but we aim at finding how certain bio-psychological types are manifested in the realm of delinquency, in the same manner as we have found these types to be manifested in various other forms of life, such as art, science, society-life, religion, recreation, etc.

In our material environmental factors such as poverty, abnormal home conditions, companions, unemployment, or unsuitable work, etc., were very conspicuous. Particularly the last-mentioned condition could be scientifically ascertained by our investigation, because we tested all the boys psychotechnically. One case may be instructive to quote :—

> *Case* 2.—Age 19 years. Tall, powerful, muscular type. Quick in his ability to sum up a position, not easily distracted in complicated mental tasks. Very good at mechanical aptitude test and can work well at machine controls with both hands. But, as so frequently occurs in these powerful muscular types, he is very weak at delicate hand or arm movements. He is not interested in delicate, artistic things ; and in a spontaneous drawing test, he drew an anvil and a heavy hammer. In the interview he informed me that he was always interested in machinery and black-smithing, but never had a chance in these directions. On the contrary, the only work he could obtain was catering on a train. This he disliked, because, as can be expected from our tests, he was totally unfit for the delicate movements and balance of crockery expected from a waiter on a train. He then worked as a labourer at £4 10s. per month. Such unskilled work for a boy with a self-assertive temperament and a good theoretical and practical intelligence, was just as unsuitable. With his calculative powers, lack of money, uninspiring work, it is very natural that he should turn to the paying concern of illegitimate liquor dealing with natives (vide Case 34 and Fig. 39).

CHAPTER II

MATERIAL AND METHODS

5. *Nature and Quantity of Material*

In the psycho-biological typology of Kretschmer with which we are mainly to deal, the adult somatic characteristics, such as hairage, muscularity, fat accumulation, anthropometrical measurements, are of primary importance. Many of these characteristics (fat, terminal hair, etc.) only start to develop after puberty, and even much later in certain instances. Although the types could to some extent be recognized before puberty, it is always better at the present stage of the typology to take subjects beyond the age of 16. We therefore considered juveniles between the ages of 16·6 years and 21·6 years only. Of these there were 105 in the juvenile adult reformatory at Tokai, and 60 and 12 in two successive investigations at Houtpoort respectively. With the aid of the Union Dept. of Prisons and the Union Dept. of Education, we investigated these boys over a period of two years by visits to the places concerned.

6. *Methods*

(a) *Interpretative Observations.*

The actual investigations proceeded in the following manner :—

The reformatory was visited by myself together with one or two well-trained post-graduate psychology students, who have had years of experience as practical teachers, to assist me. Such visits lasted from a month to two-and-a-half months.

All the inmates of the institution, upon their concurrence, were subjected to a series of psychotechnical tests, comprising mechanical aptitude, finger and manual skill, drawing, memory for forms and instructions, insight into concrete spatial relations, etc. Two to three boys were taken into the room together and given these tests individually. It took about three hours to complete each set. The social atmosphere was very free and natural, because the boys were not forced to do anything. Between actual tests they could converse with one another, sometimes enjoyed the attempts or failures of one another, and were pleased to escape the gloom of the school or workshop for a moment. Experience has taught us indubitably that the reformatory boys are strikingly suspicious in connection with strange government people who come to them. They are deeply under the impression of the detectives' activities. In one of our tests the subjects had to underline the word which they most disliked, and the word " detective " was always thickly underlined by the reformatory subjects. One of the boys asked me whether there were any secret cameras or X-rays in our apparatus. All of them thought that we were " mad doctors " (psychiatrists) who came to test them with a view to commitment to a mental institute. Accordingly, if we wanted to obtain any valuable information about their real temperaments, it was necessary to restore goodwill, mutual trust, etc. We particularly endeavoured to gain their friendship and goodwill by making jokes as we continued, about the tests themselves, such as—" Don't you think that the man who made these silly tests was an escaped lunatic ? " We repeated to them that we were no Government officials, but poor students who paid our own fares, etc. We can assert in full confidence that in most of the cases we gained their complete confidence and goodwill in the course of fourteen days. Such little incidents as handing back to them their illegal tobacco when discovered, conniving at a secret smoke, did everything to show them that we intended to be friends rather than guards over them. In their house-committee meetings, their swimming, their sport pavilion, their work, we saw them daily, and everywhere aimed at two things :

First, to obtain an all-round and intimate knowledge of their temperaments and characters, and, secondly, to foster that goodwill and emotional rapport which I deem to be necessary to know any individual. A comparison between the confessions of the boys in the interviews and the actual history as revealed by the records and Court evidence showed us that we had gained the confidence of most of them.

With regard to our first main aim, an all-round and intimate knowledge of their temperaments, we adopted the following simple method : all the observers always made short notes about every occasion on which they encountered the boy in various fields, starting with the period during which he was psychotechnically tested, to the occasion of anthropological measurements, the occasion when his photograph was taken, his general intelligence was tested and all the other systematic and casual encounters. We always placed the temperamental and character side in the foreground of our interest, but it was not done in a questionnaire form. This we did purposely, as the questionnaire is necessarily a limitation, and also this method proved less effective, in our experience, than the free characterization.[1]

Apart from these systematic encounters, we had ample opportunities to watch them at swimming, on the football field, in their debating society meetings, in their boys' court, while at work in their leisure-hour gardens, in the workshops, etc. A psychologically trained observer must, over a period of a few months of such daily contact, find innumerable opportunities to register valuable impressions. We shall offer a few out of our voluminous notes :—

(1) One of the boys has escaped. Discipline is enforced more severely. The taller boys arrange to " thrash out " secretly a few newcomers who also talk about absconding. In the recreation hour the ordeal is executed ; of the three punished one is an Athletic Pyknic—he is not the ringleader, but jumps in first to receive his " belting ". The

[1] Cf. also W. Peters, 9th Kongress f. Expt. Psychologie, 1925, p. 205. He found that a better general impression of a personality was gained from free characterizations than from a psychographic scheme.

ringleader, an Athletic Leptosome, waits to the last when the belters are tired and then gets an insignificant thrashing. We have the impulsive Pyknic versus the hesitating, calculative Leptosome.

(2) Two Catholic boys have to remove their rosaries to be anthropometrically measured. The one puts it down carefully, the other jerks it off into a corner together with his shirt. By themselves, these incidents are valueless ; in a wide series they are extremely significant.

(3) While we are testing, one of the boys outside the room spots a small wild animal creeping into a wall. A group of five go to dislocate it. A Leptosomic Athletic musters them and places each one on a point, starts with the heavy stones himself and does not worry about the safety of the smaller ones down below him. We have here the cold military type.

(4) When interviewing the boys, I placed a chair some distance from the table at which I sat. A jovial Pyknic promptly placed the chair nearer to me before seating himself, saying : " No, sir, we are going to talk together, aren't we ? " The manner in which they narrate their " stories ", in some cases very spirited, in others lamely, is from our point of view very significant. The way they greet every morning is just as significant.

(5) For photographing the boys, I had six slips ; with these were one pair of bathing knickers. One of the boys, in spite of contrary suggestions by the others, would not stand in anything else than the bathing knickers. Another boy only agreed to be photographed if taken alone. Both these boys happened to be Leptosomes (the first mentioned even had feministic somatic stigmata), and these observations therefore fit in splendidly with the reserved sensitivity of the Leptosome.

Needless to say, our observations did not always work out so perfectly at the first glance. Successive cross-sections or views of the same temperament often proved to contradict one another. The same happened in connection with observations by different observers. But in most cases we were able to explain such discrepancies as our knowledge of the cases in question increased. This point is admirably illustrated by the following example, fully described in case No. 44 (para. 35) :

My own observations were : slow and weak energy at tests ; sullen, disinterested expression ; does not associate freely with his fellows in the testroom ; inferior feelings probably ; reserved and little initiative ; fatalistic attitude when tests slightly difficult.   My colleague, however, disagreed with me, and stated that he observed the boy to be of a sociable disposition and well-liked by his fellows. My own observations at the swimming pond were : hypomanic temperament, shows much energy and talks enthusiastically.   On other occasions, too, I observed that he was boyishly frank, even mischievous at times.   His records also indicate that he is an undaunted adventurist and sexual enthusiast (gonorrhea).   The case became clear when we found out that the boy was very unpersistent and easily discouraged, especially in scholastic tasks.   He hates school, and the test room atmosphere.   The result is that, particularly before he knew us well enough, his courage in the tests almost failed him from the start.

(b) Records.

Apart from these observations, we perused all their records for past history, convictions and court procedures. We paid special attention to the methods employed in their delinquency.   The mere general types of delinquency, such as theft, burglary, etc., do not say much from a temperamental point of view.   Under certain circumstances common theft may entail more energy, optimism and daring than house-breaking and *vice versa*.[1]   The types of delinquency generally spoken of are legal or normic and not psychologically orientated types.   All such details as : the time of the day or night when a crime was committed ; whether in company or alone ; if in company, who took the lead ; the subsequent behaviour, e.g. in protecting themselves from discovery ; the quickness and completeness of confession when charged were carefully noted.

(c) Letters.

Furthermore, at Tokai we read through all the letters— approximately 700 letters—written by the boys over a

---

[1] Professor Böhmer (*Monatschrift f. Krim. Ps.*, Bd. 19, p. 207) also lays special emphasis on the wrong procedure of seeking correlations between the psycho-types and the rough divisions of crime, instead of between types and definite forms of motivation and procedures in crime.

period of two-and-a-half months, without their knowledge. The Christmas month was included in this period and proved to be very significant, because many boys received presents and delicacies, and it was generally extremely instructive to note the different attitudes taken towards " the old folk at home ". The following extracts from letters may give some idea of what we were able to glean from this heretofore somewhat neglected field of information :—

(1) *Subject R.*—Wrote nine letters in two-and-a-half months, i.e. two more than the average. *Notes made :* optimistic ; starts with clean conscience this year ; will yet make a man out of himself ; little family bits and news, in the manner of a girl away from home ; " poor daddy " ; God will keep his record clean ; encourages " ma " ; primary functioning ; swings from one emotion to the other, yet always pleasant and enthusiastic ; a woman's temperament ; hurried, irregular, yet cultured handwriting ; " I would write a long letter if I had more news " ; but will be home soon ; many X's to mother ; short sentences ; businesslike discussions about his trade—can earn £3 10s. per week (! ?) when he leaves reformatory ; pleased that Christmas over, because last at Tokai ; asks cousin to come to see him, will shave himself nicely for the occasion and pick her a fine bunch of flowers ; asks snaps ; wants to explain to her what a fool he was to abscond ; very anxious that she should come ; asks mother to come and see him ; has not heard from her for a long time ; she should come to their cricket match on Saturday ; unreflectively and emotionally religious ; prayed together with his pal every night ; asks toothpaste, handkerchiefs, soap, and razor-blades ; weak punctuation ; asks lady-friend to come and see him.

This subject happened to be a Pyknic, of the hypomanic variety, with some muscularity ; lively, full eyes and reddish face. The labile emotions, sociability, naive optimism, childlike, unreflective and spirited attitude towards life are fairly evident from his letters.

(2) *Subject S.*—Athletic Leptosome. Wrote three letters in same period. *Notes made :* intelligent ; calculating ; begins to adapt to reformatory conditions ; reasonable to brother ; need not worry about him ; wants to earn more while in custody, brother should write to authorities to get

him into a labour colony where his work is paid ; came into reformatory through bad company and no lawyer to defend his case. (In reality, he was the man who arranged everything for his companions, forged and stole cheques, etc.)

(3) Infantile Leptosome on the borderline of feeble-mindedness. *Notes made* : weak spelling ; incoherent sequence ; complains that he cannot read mother's letters ; longs for home ; rows of X's (kisses) to mother ; spells phonetically ; will buy his elder sister a doll when he comes out here ; when she marries she must send him a photograph ; extremely primitive ideas ; about calves, family, fruit ; very fatalistic religion on a low level ; will never do wrong again if only they would set him free.

(d) Experiments directly involving Temperament.

Though, as we have pointed out previously, the trained observer can glean valuable information in regard to temperaments from any task or situation presented to a subject, we have also made four experiments on the Tokai and Houtpoort boys, which are more directly related to temperamental factors :—

(*a*) We took an ergogram from each boy in the ordinary manner with a Mosso Ergograph.[1]

(*b*) The Blotpicture experiment of Rohrschach was applied to every boy.

(*c*) The Bourdon concentration test was applied to every boy.[2]

(*d*) A spontaneous drawing. Every boy was given a sheet of paper and told to draw whatever he wished, or whatever he was interested in. This method seems to be really valuable, because it entails so much spontaneity ; it is very simple— and one has to consider this point very strongly when dealing with neglected juveniles ; it indicates not only the direction of interest, but also the intro- or extraversion to a certain extent—jovial extraverted boys rarely find time to practice drawing, and if they do, the objects drawn are of a different class.

(e) Interviews.

This we consider a very important part of our investigations. As previously pointed out, we endeavoured to

[1] Skawran, *Typologie der Ergogramme.*
[2] As used by Faul, *Meteorological influences on Concentration*, Pretoria, 1931.

establish friendly relations with the boys all along. At the close of our stay, I personally interviewed each boy privately. He was told in a friendly way that everything he said was voluntary and would in no way influence his position. I flattered them by telling them that they knew themselves better than any other person, and eased them by saying that after they had been detained for such a period they could retrospect calmly and tell me " how it all happened ", " how it all started," " what was his weak point or his bad side." I knew as much as I could glean from the records, so that by tactful questioning I could direct their attention more definitely on what I considered the weak links in the chain of information (I took care that the boys did not know of my perusal of their records).

By comparing their tales with the actual crime sheets, I could convince myself that only in 5 per cent were there attempts to seriously dissimulate. In this way I obtained more particulars of the actual circumstances, and I had a view of the boys' attitude and behaviour towards parents, school, books, work, girls, bioscopes, dances, drink, society life, law and order, prison, etc., etc. The sequel must speak for itself. I continually kept a close eye on the expressions when the different phases were portrayed. I must admit that there were very few boys whom in some way or other I did not begin to like afterwards.

(f) Photographs and Anthropological Investigation.

Every boy was measured and described anthropometrically according to the scheme in the Psycho-Biogram of Kretschmer.[1] The different boys were then classified under the types as far as this was possible.[2] From these, the averages were worked out. Every individual was then

[1] Kretschmer, *Medizinische Psychologie*, Leipzig, 1930, p. 227.
[2] The author (and other collaborators of our institute) has done similar measurements and descriptions on nearly 200 Tradeschool juveniles and University students previous to the present investigation, and therefore commands the necessary experience to be able to classify boys preliminarily from their general morphological characteristics before the subtle differences in measurement are considered.

compared with the averages of his type and the pronounced exceptions reconsidered with the view to reclassifying them if necessary, or placing them aside with the indeterminable. We shall discuss the difficulties encountered in these respects when we describe the types. We need only mention here that the measurements, descriptions and photographs were studied for months with sometimes very interesting results. It is nearly impossible to get these types in a pure form, and certain exceptions in an otherwise relatively pure case frequently only become apparent after much handling.

Two views were taken of every boy with a plate camera at a distance of ten feet. These views were the direct front and the direct side (profile) view. The delinquent boys were not taken absolutely nude (vide photos in texts) because it was found that this would cause resentment on their part, leading to resistance of our investigation, frustration of the established friendly relations—so necessary for the interviews—and would also be inadvisable from a reformatory point of view. The photographs are deemed a very essential feature of our investigation. Many morphological peculiarities such as assymetries, feminisms, etc., were only detected upon careful scrutiny of each photograph.

In the anthropometrical descriptions we also paid attention to the bodily (functional) stigmata connected with the types of Jaensch, such as shine of eyes, velvety skin, tetanoid stern face with folds on forehead.[1] It is our intention to show some of the relations existing not only on the mental side, but also on the biophysical side between the types of Kretschmer and Jaensch.

7. *The Scientific Value of Interpretive Observations*

We have approached our material from a " temperament " and " character " point of view. On this account we had to make ample use of, and attached supreme importance to, interpretative or intuitive descriptive observa-

---

[1] W. Jaensch, *Grundzüge*, pp. 104, 106, 146, 150, etc.

tions in all possible situations.   Our observations have been aided fundamentally by psychotechnical experiments in so far as such experiments brought the subjects in various situations which made observation possible.   But we have not made much use of direct experimental results. This is not because we are in principle against experiments. On the contrary, we are very much in favour of psychological experiments as far as this is possible.   In fact, in our institute the typological studies have been fully supplemented by instrumental controls.[1]   Also the typological differentiations of the school of E. R. and W. Jaensch have largely been based on laboratory experiments. We have ourselves made some experiments on these delinquent boys, as we have previously shown.   But all experiments or tests must be supplemented by extensive observations describing the general attitudes (Einstellungen) and emotional responses towards the experimental situations.   W. Jaensch has criticised the typology of Kretschmer, inter alia, because it approaches its material in an intuitive, descriptive way starting from the highest mental function-layers, such as emotionality, excitability, and attitudes.[2]   W. Jaensch believes that in the layer-structure of the mind, the so-called " eidetic images " belong to a lower mental layer, i.e. are less directly (intimately) bound up with the self-conscious ego than the functions investigated by Kretschmer.   We shall later on discuss more fully the concepts of ego-consciousness, mental layers and the relations between the types of Jaensch and the types of Kretschmer.   Here we need only point out that the students of E. R. Jaensch also made extensive use of so-called " intuitive, descriptive (interpretative) observations ", to explain the typical personality structures.   E.g. Möckelmann observes that the more athletically built tetanoid type is less sociable, prefers solitude, does not easily establish emotional rapport

[1] Skawran, *Typology of Ergograms*, Pretoria, 1930.   Also F. Faul, *Meteorological Influences on the Concentration of High School Children*, Pretoria, 1930 ; G. Poggenpoel, *Psychotechnical Abilities of the Types of Kretschmer*, Pretoria, 1931.
[2] W. Jaensch, *op. cit., Grundzüge*, Berlin, 1926, p. 290.

with those he meets, is not frank and confiding, but cool, formal, and official. In fact, the real temperamental part of Möckelmann's exposition depends almost entirely on observations made on the sports-field, in conversations, at college, etc.[1] Similarly, Oeser, whose experiments on tachistoscopic reading in the Jaensch types have added substantially to the knowledge of the types, supplements his experimental findings with splendid observations of an " intuitive descriptive " nature.[2] E.g. the naive questions asked by the B-type during the experiment ; their naive self-feeling and enthusiasm expressed inter-jectionally when certain results are obtained in the experiment ; the regularity of attendance and feeling of duty of the T-type. Oeser describes the different pleasure-states in the two types with intuitive subtlety. He uses his observations to refute antagonistic views (e.g. " This idea is incompatible with the very naive, given-up-to-the-object *impression* which the integrated type creates during the experiments " [3]). Oeser also intentionally quotes Lucke, another Jaensch student, to prove the value of natural environment and conditions as found in Psychiatry, Child [4] and Animal Psychology, and the value of the interview-method and observation of the whole behaviour of subjects : " Nowhere else is the subject given in his entirety. Here, however, the experimenter not only hears words, the meaning of which he still has to interpret correctly, but here he sees from the mimicry, the eyes, the attitude, the carriage ; here he hears from the intonation and rhythm of the voice whether, and in what relation the discovered part-components are intrinsic-ally bound up with the whole personality." [5]

---

[1] H. Möckelmann, *Persönlichkeitstypus des Sportlers und Turners*, Marburg, 1929, pp. 42, 43, 49, 51, 52, and 54.
[2] Oeser, " Tachistoskopische Leseversuche " in *Zeitschrift für Psychologie*, Bd. 112, 1929, p. 161, 163.
[3] Oeser, *op. cit.*, p. 182.
[4] Cf. also, Skawran, (" Furcht und Angst in Frühen Kindesalter," *Archiv. f. d. Ges. Psycho.*, Bd. 77) who combined natural conditions with intentional experimental interference and gives his conclusions in an " intuitive descriptive " form.
[5] Oeser, *op. cit.*, p. 156.

If the typical differences in the more primitive levels, such as the typical differences between the eidetic images of the B-type, and the eidetic images of the T-type, really depend on differences of the "primitive" levels themselves, and are not due to differences of "higher" levels, such as emotions, acts of attention, attitudes, then the Jaensch school has now definitely extended the reach of these typical differences from those "lower" layers to the "higher" layers of the mind; and for the study of the higher levels, the Jaensch school now makes use of "intuitive descriptive observations", as we have just illustrated.[1] But it is still possible that the typical differences experimentally shown in the levels of the eidetic phenomena are due to influences from the top. The, in many respects, outstanding experiments of Oeser, at the institute of E. R. Jaensch, on tachistoscopic reading were essentially interpretation (Deutungs-) experiments, and as such deal largely (as he has shown) with attitudes (Einstellungen) bound up with the "highest" layers of the Ego pyramid [2] : So that Jaensch possibly did not actually exclusively handle the so-called "lower levels" of the mind when he first discovered typical differences in the eidetic images. Störring [3] has shown from pathological material that in all perception we have a fusion of images with sensations, i.e. elements from both the "higher" and "lower" levels of the mind. Skawran, [4] moreover, has illustrated that in the child mind attitude already plays a vast rôle. In practical conditions it is, therefore, hardly possible to isolate the "higher" from

---

[1] W. Jaensch also admits this (op. cit., p. 287, footnote) : "For investigation of the higher mental processes E. R. Jaensch has now evolved a combined experimental—structural—psychological procedure." The main difference between Jaensch's and Kretschmer's typology, accordingly, seems to lie in the origins ; Jaensch from the eidetic images, Kretschmer from the insanities. The one seems to be as biological as the other, because the insanities are also—even if morbid—based on biological functions, like the eidetic images. Moreover, "Basedowoid" and "Tetanoid" are methodologically just as valuable or as impeachable as "Cycloid" and "Schizoid".

[2] We shall discuss the problem of attitude more intensively in later chapters .

[3] Störring, *Psychologie*, Leipzig, 1923, p. 161.

[4] "Furcht und Angst im Frühen Kindesalter."

the " lower " if these vague distinctions may be at all permissible. Moreover, there is no evidence to prove that when the intrinsic nature of the " higher " processes is to be studied, the safest method is to trace their influences on the " lower " layers first, i.e. to start from the lower levels and work up to the higher ones. Also, as we shall show in a later chapter, it is much more possible for the bio-physiological correlates of typical differences on the emotional, impulse, and volitional side of the personality to be discovered first, because it is an acknowledged biological fact that the functions genetically earlier acquired have a smaller variability than those later acquired. The functions which Kretschmer investigated are also just as much, if not more, correlated with endocrine-vegetative-somatic conditions as the after-images and eidetic images from which Jaensch started.   W. Jaensch [1] admits that Kraus's views may be true, viz. that the type is manifested more distinctly and sharply in higher mental functions such as the nature of imagery processes.   In fact, at present the students of Marburg and W. Jaensch himself describe and expound their typological findings largely in observational interpretative terms.

As supporters of the school of Störring, who has indicated that there is no need for an additional " Understanding Psychology " apart from the present " natural-science " psychology,[2] we do not intend to advocate purely intuitive expositions based on slight verificatory evidence.   But, especially in the origination of theories as opposed to their verification, " intuitive understanding " in the typology of temperament seems to be definitely necessary. Such " understanding " must then be based on introspection studies of the investigators, if possible under experimental conditions.   Though the psychiatrist may not have been trained in this manner, he has the safe-guard of wide clinical experience, and his own inevitable introspective self-analyses.   In our case we definitely

---

[1] *Grundzüge*, p. 328.
[2] Störring, 10*th* *Kongress f. Expt. Psych*, Bonn, 1927 ; also *Geistes-wissensch'lichen und Verstehenden Psychologie*, Leipzig, 1928.

based our "interpretations" on general psychological theory. For instance, the analysis of emotions into feeling tones, organ sensations, excitement and tension, the theory of volitional attitudes which produce the active type of perseveration, and the theory of passive perseveration due to feeling states—all these theories, so lucidly exposed and adequately proved on pathological and intropective evidence by the school of Störring—have been of immense help to us in " understanding " and " interpreting " the types. It is in this respect that our studies on temperament and character differ fundamentally from those based on " enquête " (questionnaire) material as in some of the studies by the school of Heymans and Wiersma. Ordinary physicians without training in psychology cannot be expected to interpret, intuitively describe, subjects so adequately psychologically, that their descriptions can be used for a characterological theory. It is striking to note the contradictions (as we shall indicate in subsequent chapters) between observations by trained members of the school of Groningen and material collected by the " enquête " method. There may have been much of " intuitive, interpretative " conceiving of the types by Kretschmer in the beginning, but subsequent pathological and experimental psychological researches seem to admirably corroborate his theories. " The way in which relations, theories (" Ergebnisse ") are originally found, does not decide the value of a science, but the way in which these theories are verified," said Selz,[1] when he tried to show that the personality-type study does not differ essentially in its methods from the intuitive building of hypotheses in Mathematics.

At any rate, for the study of temperamental and characterological typical differences, the exclusive use of *direct* experiments at the present stage of experimental psychology seems to be neither the only reliable nor the most instructive method of gleaning information. It is altogether strange that a psychiatrist like W. Jaensch

---

[1] O. Selz, "Persönlichkeitstypen und die Methoden ihrer Bestimmung," *VIII Kongress f. Expt. Psycho*, Leipzig, 1923, p. 5.

34   CONSTITUTION-TYPES IN DELINQUENCY

should take exception to an "intuitive descriptive study of types" where this is the common method in psychiatry.[1] We fully agree that conclusions should be based on actual facts observed and that, as Stern indicates in child psychology, all the facts should be mentioned apart from the conclusions. But we cannot possibly come to the real intrinsic relations of the facts in the sense of temperaments and character, if some measure of "intuition", empathy (Einfühlung), is not used. Our observations, though largely of a descriptive nature, and dealing with emotional, impulse and volitional reactions, have been based on actual concrete facts, observations sometimes only made possible by placing the individual before a psycho-technical task. Fundamentally, therefore, there does not seem to be any difference between the present-day methods of E. R. Jaensch and ours ; also from a methodological point of view our methods do not seem impeachable.

8.   *Psycho-pathological Method*

There is another aspect of our observations and material that needs special recognition. Many of the boys are borderline cases with regard to the emotional, impulse and volitional (temperament and character) side of their personalities. The fact that they have been convicted repeatedly is proof that from a social point of view, they are abnormal. Such abnormal material forms what Störring calls "Experimente der Natur",[2] and he, together with others, as Höffding, Ziehen, Thalbitzer,[3] was one of

---

[1] Cf. the classical works of Bleuler and Bumke. A brilliant example of intuitive descriptive psychological treatment of the higher processes is to be found in Carl Schneider's *Psychologie der Schizophrenen.*

[2] *Psychologie*, p. 21.

[3] Thalbitzer, *Emotion and Insanity*, London, 1926. In the preface of this interesting work, Professor Höffding emphasizes the value of descriptive psychology, especially if aided by psychopathology. In Anglo-American psychology, this method has also been used with signal success ; Rivers, *Instinct and the Unconscious* ; J. T. MacCurdy, *The Psychology of Emotion* ; McDougall, *Outline of Abnormal Psychology.* We need not even mention the psycho-analytical school, so well known are their results in this direction.

the strongest advocates of what he terms the psychopathological method.   Some of the individual mental
processes, as Störring indicates, are abnormally accentuated
and in that way relatively isolated (abgehoben) from the
other processes, in pathological cases.   The functional
relations can accordingly be much more easily " read off ".
For the psychology of temperaments, our delinquent
material should accordingly be more valuable than normal
material.

CHAPTER III

TYPES OF PHYSIQUE [1]

The Leptosome [2]

(a) Measurements.

Skull [3] :—
Circum. 55·1.
Diam. Sagittal, 19·3.
,, Frontal, 15·2.
,, Vertical, 23·8.

Face :—
Height, 18·5.
Height of Mid-Face, 8·0.
,, Chin, 4·7.
,, Forehead, 5·8.
Length of Nose, 5·7.
Breadth at Malars 13·5.
Breadth of Lower Jaw 11·3.

Height 174. *Weight,* 60·6.

Circum. :—
Forearm, 25·2.
Calf, 32·5.
Ear to ear, 34·6.

Circum. :—
Chest, 83·3.
Stomach, 70·7.
Hips, 86·2.

Length :—
Legs : (Trochanter), 91·0.
(Ilio-spinale), 101·4.
Forearm, 28·2.
Hand, 19·6.

Breadth :—
Shoulders, 36·0.
Hips, 32·0.
Chest, 27·9.

Indices :—
Skull, 78·75.
Pignet's, 30·1.
Chest : Shoulder, 43·2.
Chest minus hips, 2·9
2 × Legs — height, 8·0.

[1] As this work deals mainly with the constitution types of Kretschmer, as described in his classical work (English translation) *Physique and Character*, London, 1925, we would recommend the reader to study this attractively written book for details and mode of measurement which, for reasons of space and the more specialized nature of our theme, we could not give in full.

[2] In the English edition (1925) this name has not yet appeared, and " Asthenic " is still used. But in his later German editions Kretschmer uses " asthenic " only for the more extreme, weak, forms (Kümmerform) of the slenderly built type. Dr. Th. van Velden (*De Bestryding van den Echtelyken Afkeer*, Leiden, 1927) takes the "leptosome" to have a fairly well developed physique as compared with the " asthenic " whom he takes to be a disease form as originally coined by Stille. We shall discuss this further in a later chapter.

[3] According to Kretschmer's Psycho-biogram, *Medizinische Psychologie*, Leipzig, 1930, p. 227, a few of the more uncommon terms may be explained thus : Skull index = (Br. × 100) ÷ Length ; Pignet's index, i.e. index of bodyfullness = height — (Chest circum. + Wt.). We may further remark that our vertical height of skull is not exactly that of Kretschmer, as it was taken from the epiglottis to the crown of the head. Our height of face = gnathion to trichion.

36

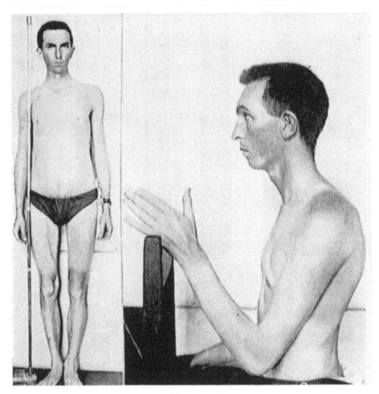

Fig. 7.

[face p. 36

From these measurements and indices and the photo-graphs of Fig. 7, 8, the following characteristics of face, skull, and body-build of the leptosome, especially as compared with the two other types, are important.[1]

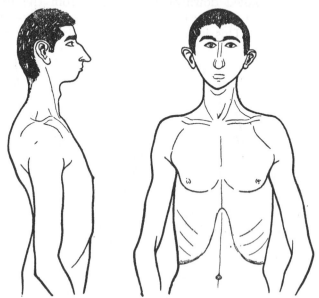

FIG. 8.—(From Kretschmer: *Körperbau und Charakter*, 1926.)

(b) *The Face,*

being according to Kretschmer, " the visiting card of the individual's whole constitution," is for diagnostic purposes very significant. The leptosome face is briefly as follows " Skin and soft parts thin, pale, poor in fat " ; skin usually stretched on bridge of nose. Bone formation of face is delicate. Very typical is the dis-proportion between the fairly long nose (compare measure-ments with those of pyknic type), and the hypoplasia of the chin and lower jaw. This is generally clearly obvious in the profile view. It results in the so-called angular profile (vide Fig. 9c, d), where the forehead is somewhat sloping and the chin receding. The lines drawn from the

---

[1] Quotations from Kretschmer, unless otherwise stated.

point of the chin to the tip of the nose, and from the tip
of the nose to the forehead, produce a clear obtuse angle.
The nose is usually thin, narrow, sharp, fairly long, if
compared with the length of the face and chin, with the
tip " rather pulled downwards ".[1] Seen from the front
such a face in pure cases has a shortened egg-shape
(vide Fig. 9g).   This is produced by the relatively broad

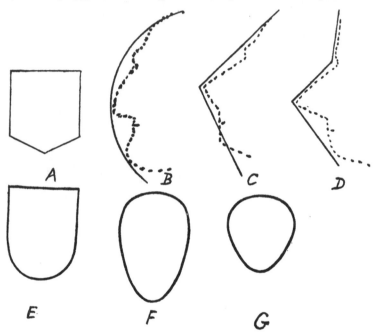

FIG. 9.—(A, E, F, G from Kretschmer : *Physique and Character*, 1926.)

forehead, hypoplastic lower jaws and lack of " fatty up-
holstering of the cheeks at the side ".   In some cases,
usually due to some athletic admixture, we find long
faces appearing longer than they really are, because of

[1] The nose in the pure leptosome is not so much pronounced because
of its real size, but, because of the receding chin and forehead, and also
because of the medium length of mid-face on which it is built.   Athletic
mixture seems to give some leptosomes a very long and large nose ;
because if one scrutinizes the more " asthenic " type (even in Kretschmer's
picture), the nose is quite medium.   The angular profile remains
characteristic of course.

their narrowness. The length is then mainly due to a longer midface (root of nose—mouth slit).

(c) The Skull.

Owing to the relative immodifiability, the skull in Kretschmer's descriptions has lost its central symptomatical value which it enjoyed in the days of Gall's phrenology. From a general point of view the skull of the leptosome may be described thus : it is small, low and of medium breadth. Kretschmer mentions that the head is usually short and the shape of the back of the head steep, showing only slight roundness. In our material, however, the steepness of the back of the skull was more obvious in athletics than in leptosomes [1] (cf. Figs. 7 and 11). Also, in our measurements we did not find the sagittal diameter to be much out of proportion as compared with the other types. Skull index of lept. = 78·75, as compared with athls. = 78·2 and pyks. = 79·9. There are also other headforms, found in leptosomes, especially when these are slightly admixed with the various dysplastic forms.

(d) General Bodybuild.

" A deficiency in thickness combined with an average unlessened length." " This deficiency apparent in all parts—face, neck, trunk, extremities and in all tissues —skin, fat, muscle, bone, and vascular system." Compare weight and circumferences with other types. On this account a relatively high Pignet's index. "A lean, narrowly-built man who looks taller than he really is." Narrow shoulders and chest if compared with measurements of hips (low index). Thin muscles, delicately boned, long arms. The chest is flat with sharp rib angle ; the belly thin, though sometimes a loose small potbelly

---

[1] Kretschmer's photographs in his main works, *Physique and Character*, *Medizinische Psychologie*, and *Geniale Menschen* (translated under the title, *The Psychology of Men of Genius*, London, 1931), do not seem to bear out his contentions on this point.

found. The leptosome, though of average height, is usually shorter than the athletic type [1] and in certain cases, especially among women, may remain relatively small. Though not mentioned by Kretschmer, I have found a tendency in the leptosome, especially in the more asthenic [2] variety to a stoop (vide photograph), while athletic admixture gives the straight vertebral column of the athletic type. There is another feature not mentioned by Kretschmer specifically, and that is the proportion of the length of the legs to the length of the rump without the neck and head. The pyknic type is described as thickset and compact (gedrungen), but the small height of the pyknic, according to my observations, is in the first place due to their short tibia-fibula bones, neck and head. We have not measured these bones separately, [3] but the length of the forearm (ulna-radius bones), corresponding to the calf-bones mentioned, according to our measurements is relatively less in pyknics than in the leptosomes and athletics (26·3, 28·1, 28·0). [4] It is notable here that these bones in the leptosome are even slightly longer than those of the athletics. From our measurements of the legs it is also apparent that the leptosomes' legs are more or less equal to those of the athletics, and a good deal longer than those of the pyknics. [5] The pyknic type accordingly has a relatively long rump and short extremities, if compared with the other types. This fact

[1] Cf. also, Skawran, *Manual of Mental and Physical Tests*, Pretoria, 1930.

[2] This tendency has also been noticed by Dr. Th. v. d. Velde (*op. cit.*, p. 255), a very careful student of constitution types.

[3] I have, however, during the last two years, specially observed these proportions. Particularly in women (where fashion has hitherto aided the anthropologist by exposing the legs), athletic or leptosomic admixture manifests very obviously in the long tibia-fibula (calf-bones).

[4] We are now investigating the relations of length of lower extremities (especially tibia-fibula) to that of the rump (symphysis-edge—sternion). It is important that the neck and head be excluded from the rump, because, according to our experience, particularly the athletic, has a "strong high neck" and also a tendency to the "high head". (Cf. also Kretschmer, *Physique and Character*, p. 48; *Medizinische Psych.*, p. 151; and Kreyenberg, *op. cit.*, p. 524.)

[5] This is also shown in the measurements of Kreyenberg (*op. cit.*, p. 521) who gives the averages for the types: lepts. 85.2; athls. 85·3; pykn.'s 83·5; and Kretschmer's own measurements (89·4, 90·9, 87·4).

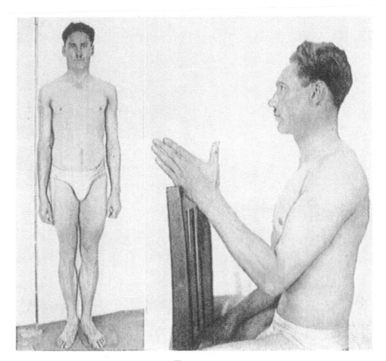

FIG. 10.

[face p. 40

has already been emphasised in a different form by the Italian school (Pende, Viola, etc.).[1] The latter especially emphasizes the importance of the rump-extremities proportion in his biotypes. Similarly, we find reference to it in the works of Professor Breitmann,[2] of Riga. These proportions seem to have very interesting biological implications, as we shall indicate in a later chapter. In measurements on a large material of epileptics by Kreyenberg, and also by Hoffmann and Delbrück, it was found that epilepsy tendencies in nearly 100 per cent

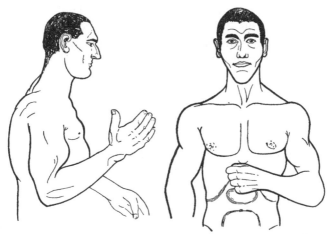

FIG. 11.—(From Kretschmer's *Körperbau und Charakter*, 1926.

of the cases go with unusual length of legs in comparison with rump-length.[3] This claims more importance if we realize that epilepsy in modern psychiatry is coming to be looked upon more and more as a bio-constitutional abnormality.[4]

---

[1] Pende, *Konstitution und Innere Sekretion*, Leipzig, 1924. We shall co-ordinate our types with these more fully in a later chapter.
[2] M. Breitmann, *Archives de Crimonologie et de Médicine Légale*, vol. i, 1927, p. 1250.
[3] Kreyenberg, *Körperbau, Epilepsie und Charakter*, p. 524.
[4] Delbrück, "Epileptisch und Epileptoid," *Archiv. f. Psych. und Nervenkrankh*, 1928, p. 708.

Mumford,[1] who has come to a similar somatic typology as that of Kretschmer apparently without any knowledge of the latter's work, describes the leptosome type as the "test tube" build. This is in accordance with our measurements which indicate narrow shoulders, chest, waist, and hips. The breadth of the hips in some cases is somewhat pronounced in proportion to the shoulders if compared with pure male-cases in the other two types. Mumford compares this type with the "wineglass" type which corresponds to certain members of Kretschmer's athletic type, viz. the broad shoulders (rim of wineglass) with relatively narrow hips (base of wineglass). Thirdly, Mumford has his "barrel" type, the compact pyknic physique of Kretschmer. (Mumford's energy descriptions also tally to some extent with what we shall outline later on.[2])

(f) *Physical Power.*

The weak muscularity and strength of the leptosome also become evident from measurements taken by us on a few hundred juveniles with a dynamometer.[3] Grip pressure : lepts. = 31·6 ; athletics = 37·0 ; pyknics = 31·5. Pulling with arms across chest : lepts. = 19·3 ; athletics = 26·04 ; pyknics = 22·3 (all in kilograms). These measurements may, in many instances, help to indicate athletic admixture in an otherwise relatively pure leptosome. The physical energy we shall touch upon in a later chapter.

(g) *Skin and Hairage.*

The skin is thin, poor in fat, and of a medium to fine texture ; not very elastic, weakly circulated.[4]

---

[1] A. Mumford, *Healthy Growth*, Oxford, 1927, p. 179.

[2] As Dr. Phaler (*System der Typenlehre*, Leipzig, 1929) remarks, the similarity of types reached by various authors in various parts of the world and from very different points of approach, is a sure proof of the validity of these developing typologies.

[3] For further particulars, Skawran, *Manual of Mental and Physical Tests*, Pretoria, 1930.

[4] The skin of Schizo's is similar to that of Jaensch's T-type—one of the proofs that there is a close relationship between the two typologies.

The hairage is very characteristic and important. We have to differentiate between primary hair and secondary hair. The primary hair of the child consists of the hair of its head, brows, and the almost invisible lanugo hairy covering of the rest of the body. At puberty is added the secondary hair: genital and armpit hair, beard, hair on the trunk, also gradual change of the lanugo hair of the extremities into secondary hair. Only the pubes and the hair under the armpits develop ordinarily before the age of 17. Accordingly, in our juvenile material, beards and hair on the chest were generally weakly developed in all types. This proved a severe handicap in diagnosing the types. The same applied to fat accumulation as we shall indicate later on.

The leptosome often has an excessive formation of head hair, not only very dense but " grows far down the neck and also inwards over the forehead and temples " ; " brows often partake in this excessive growth ". The individual hairs are usually thin but have a tendency to stand erect. Such profuse, thin, straight head hair may be called " Fur cap " hair in Kretschmer's terms (vide Fig. 7, 31). This kind of thin, erect standing " fur " hair is a very important characteristic, which Kretschmer has not emphasized sufficiently. Leptosomes can be differentiated from athletics in this respect. The athletic's hair, though also straight (not erect), is much coarser in fibre, and generally in proportion to the athletic's more robust build. There is much less tendency in leptosomes and athletics to become bald than in pyknics, and if they do, the bald patch is usually irregular and with a matt surface, as compared with the shining bald heads of pyknics. The lanugo hair over the body often is also well-grown. The secondary hair of the leptosome, contrary to the primary hair just described, is much less developed. Weak beard, mostly localized in front of ears, on chin and upperlip (Chinese beard). Armpit and genital hair medium (if no dysplastic influences—infantilisms and eunuchoidism). Scanty hair on chest.

10. The Athletic Type [1]

(a) Measurements.

Skull :—
    Circum., 56·2.
    Diam., Sagittal, 19·7.
        ,,   Frontal, 15·4.
        ,,   Vertical, 24·4.

Face :—
    Height, 18·7.
    Height of Mid-face, 8·4.
        ,,   Chin, 4·9.
        ,,   Forehead, 6·1.
    Length of Nose, 5·85.
    Br. at Malar Bones, 13·9.
    Br. of Lower Jaw, 11·6.

Weight, 70·4.   Height, 176·0.
Circum. :—
    Forearm, 27·0.
    Calf, 35·0.
    Ear to ear, 35·2.

Circum. :—
    Chest, 91·0.
    Stomach, 76·0.
    Hips, 92·1.

Length :—
    Legs : (Trochanter), 90·3.
           (Ilio-spinale), 100·1.
    Forearm, 28·0.
    Hand, 19·6.

Breadth :—
    Shoulders, 38·3.
    Hips, 33·0.
    Chest, 29·6.

Indices :—
    Skull, 78·2.
    Pignet's, 14·6.
    Chest, Shoulders, 42·1.
    Chest, Hips,-1·1.
    2 × Legs — Height, 4·6.

(b) Similarities with Leptosomes :—

In describing the main features of the leptosome we have made several comparisons with the other types. Also in Kretschmer's descriptions, the leptosome and the athletic, both belonging to the Schizothyme-Schizoid-Schizophrene series, are shown to have also many somatic constitutional features in common, e.g. weak fat accumulation ; tallness ; length of legs ; long faces ; angular profiles ; profuse primary hair ; disinclination to regular, shiny, bald heads ; hair straight as compared with the soft wavy hair frequently found in the pyknic ; pale colour of skin, etc. We may, therefore, describe the athletic type more cursorily, and indicate his special characteristics only.

(c) Face and Skull.

On a powerful high neck is seated a coarse " highhead ", with a high middleface and firm powerful trophism of the bones and skin ; well-defined supra-orbital arches ;

---

[1] Only to retain uniformity we would accept this name because " athleticism " in the English sense seems to be an aptitude of the athletic leptosome rather than the extreme muscular type.

" a projecting, well-moulded chin " ; a snub nose, often very large. In the classical case the profile-line (i.e. line joining tip of nose to forehead and tip of chin respectively) shows a gentle curve mainly due to the high nose being counteracted by the projecting chin ; but many instances of angular profiles and large-nosed profiles are also found. The frontal view gives an elongated egg-shape (Fig. 9f), due to the " length-wise hyperplasia of the mid-face and chin ". According to our measurements the head is of medium size, usually steep at the back.

(d) Bodybuild.

Usually tall (compare height measurements) ; particularly broad, projecting shoulders, a superb chest, and a trunk characterized by a strong development of the skeleton, musculature and skin. The heavily built shoulders in comparison with a proportionate pelvis and hips gives the " wineglass " impression of Mumford. But our measurements show that the heavy bone trophism usually leads to heavy hip-bones as well (cf. also the measurements of Kretschmer and Kreyenberg). The extremities also show heavy bones and joints well proportioned by the plastic muscle relief. The free neck with the " sloping linear contour of the firm trapezius " gives this part of the shoulders, if viewed from the front, its very characteristic form.

(e) Skin and Hairage.

The skin of the athletic we found to be thick, firm and with a characteristic coarse texture. This texture contrasts very typically with the fine texture of the soft, velvety skin of the pyknic.[1] The head hair of the athletic is usually straight (not erect) and hard. The beard is more developed than that of the leptosome but less than the dense and well-distributed beard of the pyknic. (Dysplasias, however, are very common in my material.)

---

[1] This is one of the instances where there is remarkable somatic correspondence between the Schizothyme and the T-type of Jaensch ; and the Cyclothyme and the B-type on the other hand (W. Jaensch, *Grundzüge*, p. 107).

After the 25th year of age the chest is, in a triangular form in the centre, inclined to be well covered with secondary hair.

II. *The Schizothyme-Schizoid-Schizophrene Group*

It is to the great merit of Kretschmer that he has both statistically and temperamental-characterologically indicated the relations between the leptosomic, athletic and dysplastic constitution and the Schizo-personality. Without committing ourselves to his theory that Schizophrenia is a mere caricature of the normal Schizo-personality,[1] we may still profit enormously by accepting Kretschmer's classical analyses of the pre- and post-psychotic Schizo-personality. We need only remember always that particularly in the postpsychotic personality Kretschmer may have struck upon characteristics which actually belong to the disease as a " process "[2] super-imposed upon the real prepsychotic personality and do not actually constitute an intrinsic development of that personality. As we have already indicated, there are on the somatic side many general trophic principles which govern the features of both the leptosomic and athletic constitution, the most obvious being : strong primary hair with weak secondary hair ; absence of fat, roundness and compactness ; long extremities ; well-developed noses often producing the characteristic angular profile ;

[1] The connection placed by Kretschmer between the Schizo-personality and the actual Schizophrenic disease process is being severely criticised by very famous psychiatrists, e.g. Bumke, *Lehrbuch der Geisteskrank-heiten*, Munchen, 1929 ; Carl Schneider, *Psychologie der Schizophrene*, Leipzig, 1930 ; Jaensch, *Grundzüge* . . ., Berlin, 1926. Also Professors Lange, Grühle, and Wilmanns also reject the main part of this theory. In spite of this, his analyses are extensively quoted. The whole problem is well outlined by L. Polen, " Körperbau und Charakter," *Archiv. f. d. Ges. Psycho.*, Bd. 66, pp. 1–116.

[2] Professor Kurt Schneider, *Die Psychopathische Persönlichkeiten*, Vienna, 1928, wants to differentiate between the personality " develop-ment ", which he views with Jaspers as an "understandable becoming", on the one hand, and the psychotic "process" as in form and contents something new and, from the personality-dispositions side, "incompre-hensible " and "inappreciable " (nicht nacherlebar) (p. 6, 7) on the other hand.

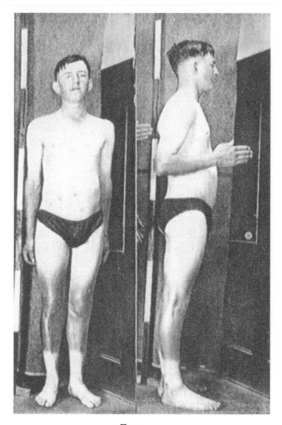

FIG. 12.

[face p 46

deep-set eyes without much lustre.[1] But it is obvious that somatically there are very distinct differences, too, between leptosomes and athletes, such as coarseness of head hair, muscularity, bones and joints, etc. We shall endeavour to show in the sequel that these differences seem to correspond to different endocrine and other biological radicals, and also to appreciable differences on the psychical side.[2] The dysplastics as a group and the various subgroups may be separately studied

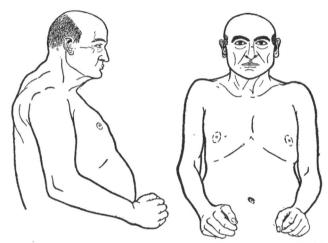

FIG. 13.—(From Kretschmer : *Körperbau und Charakter*, 1926.)

[1] Kretschmer mentions only cursorily, when discussing the pyknic constitution, that they sometimes have exopthalmia, but more often small deep-set eyes. We have, however, in normal material constantly found the eyes of pyknics to be fairly large, bright, youthful, and shallow-set—even *protusio bulborum*. The eyes of other types where pyknic admixture is absent, were found to be deep-set and without the bright youthful lustre of that of the pyknic (cf. Figs. 7, 40). The same impression is created when the photographs in Kretschmer's books are carefully studied. We shall return to this when discussing the relations of our typology with that of W. Jaensch, and the biophysiological bases of these types. The B-type of Jaensch has such bright protruding youthful eyes.

[2] Kretschmer, himself, also gradually starts to outline more differentiated correlations between the psychical subtypes and the somatic subtypes (cf. Enke, *Zeitschrift f. Ang. Ps.*, Bd. 36, pp. 237–87 ; and Kretschmer, " Biologische Persönlichkeits-diagnose in der Straf-rechtspflege," *D. Jur. Zeitung* 31, p. 783). In his original work, the main aim was the relations between the Schizo-personality as a whole, and the physique types to which it has a biological affinity.

from the psychological and psychopathological side as well, in order to find more differentiated correlations between biophysical constitutions and psychological types.[1]

12. The Pyknic Type

(a) *Measurements.*

Skull .—
Circum., 55·5.
Diam., Sagittal, 19·4.
,,   Frontal, 15·5.
,,   Vertical, 23·8.

Face :—
Height, 18·5.
Height of Mid-face, 8·0.
,,   Chin, 4·7.
,,   Forehead, 6·3.
,,   Nose, 5·5.
Br. at Malar Bones, 14·0.
Br. of Lower Jaw, 11·9.

Height, 167·0.   *Weight,* 62·5.

Circum. :—
Forearm, 25·8.
Calf, 34·0.
Ear to ear, 35·2.

Circum. :—
Chest, 87·5.
Stomach, 70·4.
Hips, 88·0.

Length :—
Legs : (Troch.), 86·5.
    (Ilio-Sp.), 96·0.
Forearm, 26·4
Hand, 19·1.

Breadth :—
Shoulders, 36·0.
Hips, 31·3.
Chest, 28·5.

Indices :—
Skull, 79·9.
Pignet's, 17·0.
Chest, Shoulders, 41·2.
Chest, Hips, -·5.
2 × Legs — Height, 6·0.

(b) *Classification difficulties of young Pyknics.*

In the juvenile material we had to deal with it was found extremely difficult to classify the pyknics adequately for the following reasons :—

(1) At this age, heterogeneous elements in the constitution come out very clearly.[2]
(2) The typical pyknic fat of the trunk usually only begins to show clearly after the 25th or 30th year of age.
(3) The secondary hair, such an important diagnostic symptom field, is also very far from its full growth between the ages of 16·6 and 21·6 years.

[1] This further differentiation is, to some extent, also attempted by Kreyenberg ; and also Mezger (*Mitteilungen*, p. 26) suggests that " special types " be built out of the dysplastics. In all such correlations between morphological-physiological and psychological qualities we emphatically do not mean single features in the sense of Lavater and Gall, but broad constitutional complex-units on the physical side with fundamental characteristics as e.g. the mood and excitement proportions, on the mental side.
[2] *Physique and Character,* 1925, pp. 52, 33.

We shall therefore describe the typical pyknic constitution more on the adult model (vide Fig. 13) and according to the works of Kretschmer.[1]

We then get the following picture :—

(c) *Face and Skull.*

The face has a tendency to " breadth, softness, and rotundity ". The skull is large, round, broad, fairly deep (sagitally), but not very high (cf. measurements). The skin has a tendency to redness on the cheeks and nose, but otherwise, has a yellowish colour. The face is the real " full-moon " type, being round with a good overlay of fat and without projecting bony structure (*vide* Fig. 12). But the plastic features and folds (e.g. the nose—lips crease) are well-formed in spite of the absence of differentiating bones.[2] The profile line is only gently curved because of the protruding domed forehead and projecting chin. The nose, moreover, is small to middle-size, a fleshy and even thick tip, blunt, often with wide nostrils and sometimes with a depressed bridge. The forehead is broad, domed, and much more prominent than in the other types : very remarkable is the similarity between the forehead of the male pyknic, the normal female and the infant in this respect.[3] At the back the

[1] We deem it necessary, if a complete knowledge of these types is required, especially with regard to peculiar forms and mixed types, to consult Kretschmer's works.

[2] Kretschmer's depiction of the pyknic—as compared with the other types—bodily as well as mentally—is very sympathetic and flattering indeed ; so much so, that at our institution the impression was created that Kretschmer must belong to this type himself. Cf. also Dr. Pfahler on this point.

[3] This is not mentioned by Kretschmer, but our observations have convinced us that there are many very interesting similarities between the pyknic build and that of any infant. Also, there are many similarities between the bodily features of the " sexually well differentiated " normal woman and the infant. This fact has also been emphasized by anthropologists generally, and Gunther (*Rassenkunde.*, München, 1929, p. 30, 118, 169) who indicates the similarity between the Alpinic racial characteristics and the pyknic constitution, mentions in his descriptions of the Alpinics the following : " In the Alpinic race, the male skull is scarcely, and often not at all, different from the female skull." He mentions further, in discussing sex-differences generally : " The female skull stands in all races somewhat nearer to the infant skull than does the male skull, because the female skull's development is ended off earlier

head, though rounded, shows but little protrusion, and it connects up directly with the short thick neck.[1] Viewed from the front the face gives the " flat five-cornered " or the " broad shield " shape (vide Fig. 9 *a*, *e*).

(*d*) *Body-build*.

" Pronounced development to the outside of the breast and stomach ; tendency to fat accumulation more on the trunk, neck and lower face than on the limbs. Height medium to small, soft broad face on a short massive neck sitting between the shoulders." Paunch protruding, and chest vaulted. Muscles not showing the relief of that of the athletic type, and usually softer. Skeleton and joints medium to delicate. Hands rather short and wide. Shoulders in the pure case are less broad than those of the athletics, but broader than those of the leptosome. Kretschmer mentions that, especially among older pyknics, the upper portion of the spinal column takes on a light kyphotic bend making the shoulders drop forwards and downwards over the swelling chest. The extremities are short, especially if compared with the length of the rump (excluding neck and head).

(*e*) *Skin and Hairage*.

We have mentioned that the pyknic usually has a good complexion over cheeks and nose. The skin, generally,

than that of the male. In all races the female has a rounder forehead (rund-stirniger) than the male . . ." " On the whole, the forehead part of the female skull is more pronounced than in the male skull . . ." " The male forehead is more strongly receding." He points out that even in the Nordic race (our leptosome with athletic admixture) the typical female profile is less angular than the male profile. The angularity of the Nordic female face with a steep forehead is then more of the type D in Fig. 9, called by Skawran the " Fourie-profile ". We shall deal fully with these interesting biological-anthropological comparisons in a later chapter.

[1] The B-type of Jaensch, which seems to correspond in essentials with the pyknic-cyclothyme type of Kretschmer, also has " a tendency to a thick neck " (Ewald, *Konstitution und Charakter*, Leipzig, 1928, p. 60). This is noteworthy because the thick neck is very characteristic in the pyknic. Kretschmer does not mention the weak development of the back of the skull in pyknics. We have, however, found this repeatedly, and it is also manifest from the photographs of Kretschmer and of Lenz.

as far as our material goes, seems to have a creamy olive tendency. On the back of the hands we find the characteristic soft, tough, fine-textured, velvety skin, with an attractive creamy olive colour. The general principle of hairage in the pyknic type is relatively weak primary (head and lanugo), with well-developed secondary (beard, chest, pubes, etc.) hair. The head hair in pure cases inclined to be soft and often wavy. The hair does not grow down over the face, but leaves a good forehead (vide measurements), and in older material bald heads of a regular shiny type are frequent. The brows often do not join over the base of the nose. Beard—important diagnostically—remarkably evenly distributed with fairly wide boundaries and somewhat dense growth. Pubes, armpits and chest hair well developed.

13. *Special Dysplastic Types*

(a) *General.*

Kretschmer places this heterogeneous group of types alongside the leptosomic and athletic types as constitutions showing a biological affinity to Schizophrenia, and in this manner to the Schizo-personality generally. They are less common in normal material but as they seem to be intimately related with glandular-dysfunctions, we should expect them to be of more importance in such borderline subjects as psychopathy, criminality, feeble-mindedness, etc.[1] These phrases describe them generally :

---

[1] In Kretschmer's pathological material, 34 out of 260 were dysplastics and all of them Schizophrenes. Kreyenberg (*op. cit.*) has shown that more or less half of his 700 epileptics were dysplastic or had striking dysplastic features. The degenerative stigmata that Lombroso indicated to be more prevalent in severe criminals would also largely fall under dysplasias. The more popular works of Carl Huter also locate mental abnormalities in so-called disharmonic constitutions. The comprehensive investigation of Dr. Goring (*The English Convict, A Statistical Study*, 1913—quoted by Burt, *op. cit.*, p. 209), however, seems to have proved that there are no more " anomalies of physique " in criminals than in normals. As previously stated, Lombroso mainly emphasized signs of degeneracy and, if Goring had not acted under this "isolated stigmata " attitude, but considered such wide constitutional anomalies as infantilisms, feminisms, masculinisms, dysglandular fat growths, etc.,

" They form striking digressions from the average " ;
" such forms of growth as vary very markedly from the
average and most common form of the types " ; " they
impress the laity as rare, surprising and ugly."

These types have by no means been adequately
described thus far, so that especially in juvenile material,
it is sometimes extremely difficult to distinguish between
them and mixtures of the main types. The following are
some of the main dysplastic groups with which we came
into contact :—

(b) The Elongated Eunuchoids and Intersexual Physiques

Extreme length of extremities in relation to the height
of the body.   A-sexual pelvis in males, or sometimes
unusual width of hips as compared with the shoulders,
and the generously curved contour of the hips which,
together with the graceful waist makes a distinct feminine
impression (*vide* Figs. 14 right, 27, 22).   Other feminine
characteristics frequently observed parallel with or apart
from the feminine waist and pelvis in the male are :
characteristic   ruddy   complexion   complicated   with
extreme aptitude to blush, soft skin, soft sentimental
eyes, high pitch of the voice, straight hair line from ear
to ear over forehead without the masculine indentations
on sides, head hair going low down in neck,[1] scanty puberty
hair with a characteristic feminine localization of the

he might have come to a different result.   Taking only under- and over-
development into consideration as possible causes of delinquency, Burt
has found 12 per cent of his male cases where these conditions figures
as " probable factors ".   That constitutional anomalies based primarily
on neuroglandular dysfunctions will be more frequent in delinquents
than in normals is, I think, a parallel condition to the frequency of
psychopathy in delinquency (vide XIII, above).   The fact that Michel
(*op. cit.*, p. 86) found experimentally extreme disturbance of pain
sensibility in 67 per cent of his 302 severe recidivists is certainly
significant.   He also found abnormally many cardiovascular anomalies.
Also Birnbaum (*op. cit.*, p. 6) mentions that bodily constitutional
anomalies are more frequent in criminals than in normals.   Thus far
this issue was prejudiced immensely by the fact that investigators
were looking for a homogeneous group in criminals rather than simply
to investigate with a view to finding all diverse constitutional anomalies.
Kretschmer himself (*D. Jur. Zeitung* 31, *Jahr.*, p. 787) believes dysplastics
to occur much more frequently in criminals than in normal people.

[1] A. Lenz, *Grundriss der Kriminalbiologie*, p. 116.

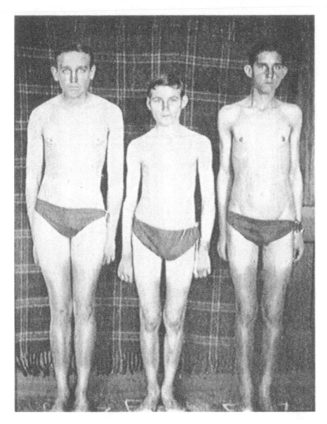

Fig. 14. Asthenic reacting types. Feminine, infantile, and
asthenic physique, resp.

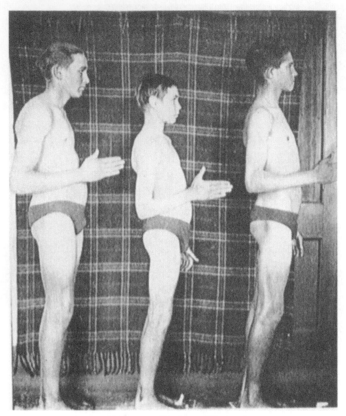

FIG. 15. (Same as Fig. 14.)

[*face p.* 53

genital hair. I also believe to have observed that the chest and abdominal parts of feministic types make a feminine impression if viewed in profile, and that the trapezius muscles are attached to the shoulders further away from the neck, producing a gradual slope from the neck towards the tips of the shoulders (vide Fig. 14 right, 23). Forward bending (kyphosis) of the upper spine, I have also noticed frequently.

From these descriptions, it becomes obvious that there are some similarities between the leptosomic physique and these intersexual types. In cases where the legs are not excessively long, or the feminine characteristics very pronounced, they may be conveniently taken as a subgroup of the leptosomic type.[1] But in many cases the intersexual factors are connected with dysplastic-athletic factors and must then be considered in that fairly different arrangement (*vide* Figs. 22, 23) (Masculinism in women is also considered a dysplasia by Kretschmer. We have not studied women delinquents and these therefore do not concern us here.)

(c) Infantilism and Hypoplastics.

All-round hypoplasia leads to a kind of miniature edition. This I found in pyknics as well as in leptosomes and athletics. They were fairly proportionately built, but in all respects on a small scale (vide Figs. 16, 17, 18). I think that in the few cases which I found there is also something of a mental parallelism which points in the direction to be expected from a study of the normal types to which they correspond—only more infantile. We shall discuss this when dealing with the mental side of the typology.

I have further found instances where not only the size constituted a deviation from the normal, but also— or even mainly—the headform, secondary hair, develop-

---

[1] We shall further discuss this fact in a later chapter. The eunuchoid as well as the leptosome is intimately connected with the status thymico Lymphaticus according to Peritz, *Innere Sekretion*, Berlin, 1923; also Berman, *Glands Regulating Personality*, New York, 1928.

ment of the nipples, or facial form and expression, made a markedly infantile or primitive appearance (vide Figs. 20, 21 centre), especially if the age was considered. There seems to be a discrepancy between the physiological and the chronological age or between certain factors in the physiological development and the real age.

Such infantilisms in shape or size, or both, may occur in certain constitutional sub-parts only, while the rest of the body constitution seems better developed, e.g. absence only of secondary hair, or hypoplastic facial proportions, etc; though here, as in all other symptom fields, it is disastrous only to go on isolated symptoms. In our cases we were almost always able to indicate various other dysplastic features together with the at first apparently isolated hypoplasias. Some such disproportionate trophisms are found in the following types:—

> (1) Hypoplastic face type, where one finds insufficient modelling of prominent parts, such as mouth, lips, and chin; eyes deep-set, piercing and, due to the insignificant nose, too near together.
> (2) Acromicria, i.e. " an elective hypoplasia of the limbs, e.g. hands and feet ". In such cases, the limbs from the knee and elbow downwards become disproportionately small and delicate. What makes this development more striking is that if often occurs in well-developed shoulders and physique generally.

In figure 19 we have something of acromicria. If we examine this individual carefully, however, we discover other dysplasias as well, e.g. the lower part of the face shows a marked hypoplasia; the lower part of the body, the flat chest and asthenic build (generally slight musculature, absence of fat, long bones, thin joints), is out of all proportion with the broad shoulders. His armpit-hair is slight, genital hair weak and localized, and at the age of 19 there is no sign of a beard or moustache! The skin is of a very fine texture. It will be instructive to compare some of his measurements with those of the average leptosome type, to which he is the nearest related (averages given in parentheses) :—

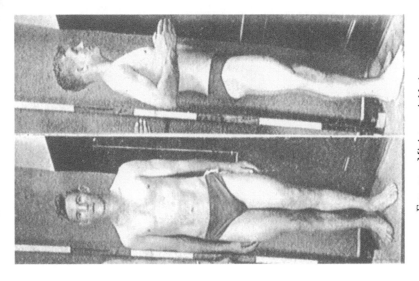

Fig. 16. Miniature Leptosome.

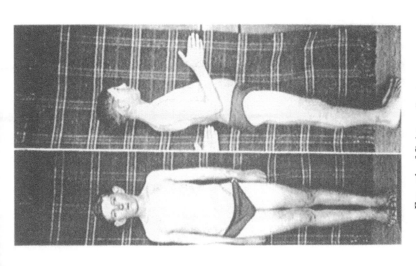

Fig. 17. Miniature Athletic.

[face p. 54

[face p. 55

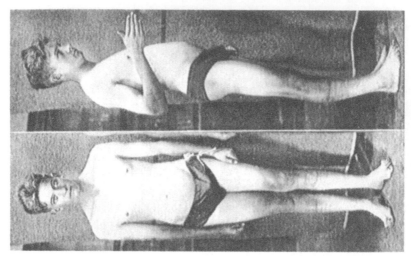

FIG. 19.   Acromicria.

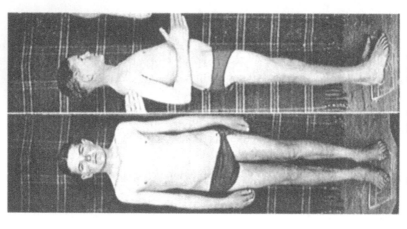

FIG. 18.   Miniature Pyknic.

Width of shoulders, 37·3 (36·0) ; of chest, 27·6 (27·9) ; of hips, 31·1 (32·0).

Height of mid-face, 7·4 (8·0) ; of chin, 4·3 (4·7) ; of body, 167 (174).

Circumference of skull, 57·5 (55·1) ; overhead from ear to ear, 35·5 (34·6) ; of chest, 85·0 (83·3) ; of hips (trochanter), 83·5 (86·2) ; of forearm, 24·0 (25·2) ; of calf, 29·0 (32·5).

Length of legs, 85·0 (91·0) ; of hand, 17·2 (19·6).

Pignet's index, 27·3 (30·1).

These measurements show more mathematically : the very broad shoulders ; normal chest ; under-developed hips (if we compare the distances of the trochanter and the ilio-spinale from the ground, 85·0 and 94·5, we get the impression that the pelvis crest bones (ilia) have not diverged sufficiently at the top, and have grown upwards instead of outwards) ; hypoplastic lower face in spite of a large skull ; weak bodyfullness—even if compared with the leptosomes, the thinnest of the types—which is in strange disproportion to his shoulders. His hands are excessively small, and from the figure this can be seen of the feet, too.

We have dealt with this case fairly exhaustively, in order to indicate the following points very emphatically :—

Firstly, dysplastic features cannot be considered as isolated stigmata, or degenerate stigmata in the sense of Lombroso. But the proportions must be considered and various additional dysplasias in all the constitutional features must be looked for.

Secondly, it shows the value of measurements to act as a check on the trained visual observative powers.

Thirdly, it stresses the value of photographs.

Fourthly, as we shall see in the mental part, extremely interesting correlations between mental constitution and bodily constitution can be discovered.

(d) *Fat Abnormalities.*

Such strong fat accumulations of dysglandular nature differ from the pyknic fat which is usually confined to the lower face, neck and trunk (belly). Polyglandular or dysplastic fat would, for example, be an isolated layer of fat round the buttocks, or over the crest of the pelvis bone (vide Fig. 46). Sometimes the whole body is encased in a diffuse layer of fat, together with plump features, coarse head hair, weak beard, etc. In some instances I found exceedingly soft, childlike head hair together with the weak beard. Various dysplastic features usually occur together and in this way the diagnosis is facilitated. But in juveniles, where the secondary hair cannot be too seriously considered and the facial and bodily features are not yet adequately differentiated, I sometimes found considerable difficulties in distinguishing between these fat dysplastics and pyknics with athletic admixture (vide Figs. 46, 44 and cases 60, 61).

(e) Athletic Dysplastics.

There are many transitions from athletics to dysgland-ular builds.[1] Such types usually retain the heavy bones, broad shoulders, and muscular powers of the athletic. But they vary in all directions from the characteristic proportionality, tallness and straightness of body, prominent facial features, etc., of the athletic. Ill-proportion and plumpness are their outstanding characteristics. Kretschmer says : " All proportions are ugly, massive, clumsy ; the skin is pasty and some-times obscured by diffuse fat-layers." We have in some of these variants also noticed a forward bend of the upper spine (kyphosis) and occasionally very weakly developed secondary hair. It is possible that feminine or intersexual constitutional factors also play a rôle here ; because kyphosis of the upper spine, peculiar attachment of the trapezius muscles to the tips of the shoulders, localization of genital hair, and forehead hair-line seem to have some connection with Mathes intersexual women and with feminine males generally. On the mental side also, hysterical and feminoid characteristics could be found in some of these (vide Figs. 22 and 23). Some of these ill-proportioned, yet strong, rugged builds also seem to

[1] Kretschmer, *Physique and Character*, p. 26. Kreyenberg in his study of 700 epileptics has also found numerous dysplasias in epileptic athletics.

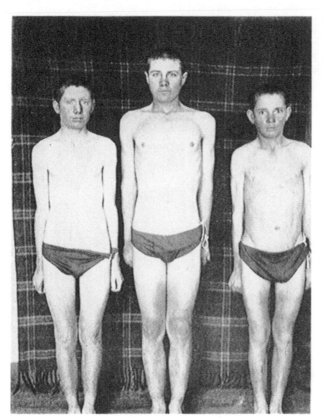

Fig. 20. Infantilisms (ages 16-17 years).

[*face p.* 56

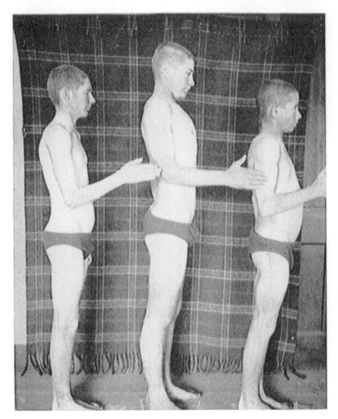

FIG. 21. (Same as Fig. 20.)

[*face p.* 57

incorporate infantile factors in their constitutions. Such infantile traits are frequently seen in the peculiar head and facial forms (vide Fig. 21 centre), and also in infantile levels of development (enuresis, etc.).

Apart from these tall, massive, big-boned athletic dysplastics we have found other variants, or perhaps types of their own, who are so short and muscularly thick-set that it is sometimes difficult to distinguish them from athletic-pyknic mixtures. In fact, we have generally experienced much difficulty in distinguishing all the plump dysplastic athletics from athletic pyknic mixtures, and we feel sure that this is undoubtedly an important source of error in classifications according to Kretschmer's typology. We have got much help from the following principles of division : the skin of these plump athletic dysplastics is pasty, matt and coarse of texture, whereas pyknics have a velvety, soft, clean and finely-textured skin. The eyes of pyknics are more protruding, large and spirited (Basedowoid). A very important differentiating principle is also the coarseness of fibre and straightness of hair which are very pronounced in these types if compared with the soft, flat-lying, often wavy hair of pyknics. The relative length of the legs and rump is another significant differentiating point in this respect.

Especially in our juvenile material we have frequently found the dysglandular, pasty fat-layer missing and then they are still more easily confused with well-trained muscular pyknics, unless the skin, hair, eyes, length of legs and trunk, etc., are also considered. This more lean group of short, ill-proportioned athletics or dysplastics gives somewhat the following impression : heavy growth of coarse-fibred head hair reaching low down the neck and the forehead, producing a low square forehead. Relatively broad shoulders and long legs if compared with the trunk. Matt, coarse skin, sometimes giving the impression of a small-pox face, thick lips (Figs. 25, 24 left).

The " Tower-skull " frequently found in the athletic group is perhaps also a dysplastic variant. It is characterized by a cone-shaped skull, under which "sits a very long, bony face with a prominent snubnose having a sharp depression at the root"; brush-like, strong beard, and bushy hair; tall, ill-proportioned body.

14. *Mixtures of Types*

Kretschmer constantly admits that mixtures between the types are perhaps just as frequent as relatively pure cases. This condition also obtains with regard to the types of Jaensch and the other biotypes. In fact, it is a condition prevalent throughout nature.[1] We know to-day that we hardly find a pure male or pure female constitution. There are innumerable grades of transition from the one to the other. The very term "type" stands for a relative pronouncement of a hierarchy of qualities which is not definitely and absolutely demarcated from all other possible pronouncements of quality-hierarchies. The one type is separated from, and merges into the other, like one hill into the other, with a wide shallow dale in between.[2] It has been pointed out that this state of affairs makes the Kretschmer typology (and all other biotypologies) unsuited for practical application in delinquency. This must certainly be admitted, but a purely psychological division of types suffers from the same fault and, moreover, has the disadvantages that the additional information to be gleaned from the physical constitution for a pure psychological typology is lost. Moreover, as long as we keep this fact of possible mixtures in mind, and exercise the necessary precautions, the very mixtures become vastly interesting. We shall see in the sequel how interesting for delinquency such mixtures as athletic-pyknic, leptosome and athletic, etc., become. We should think of the types not in the form of pigeon-holes, but in positions on a scheme such as my proposed "Triangle of Temperaments" (vide para. 58, Figs. 50, 51).

[1] Professor Fetscher, *Mitteilungen der Krim. Biol. Ges.*, 1928, p. 39.
[2] Wm. Stern, *Differentielle Psychologie*, 1921, Leipzig, p. 168.

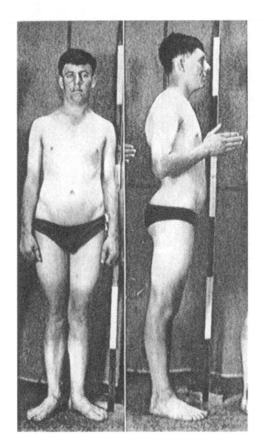

FIG. 22.

[face p. 58

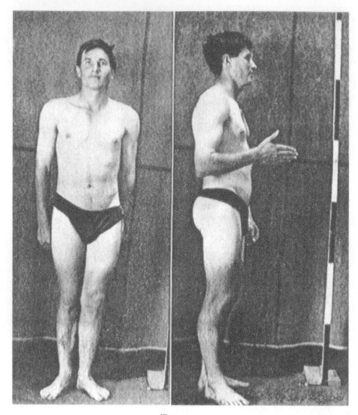

FIG. 23.

[face p. 59

In this way, mixtures will assist a more subtle differentiation of sub-types both on the physical and mental sides. It is by comparing various mixtures with one another, in regard to specific constitutional, and various other dysglandular, vegetative and neural features, that we can eventually reach more differentiated correlations between the mental and physical sides of the constitution.

We find all possible sorts of mixtures. Pyknic head and shoulders on athletic length of legs (vide Fig. 44); small leptosome skull on something of a. pyknic face (beard and roundness, profile line) and trunk, and perhaps again, leptosome legs ; pyknic roundness and fat with very strong and heavy muscles ; pyknic face and body lines with pronounced width of shoulders, etc. The training necessary to observe and describe all these characteristics adequately only comes with long practice, as Kretschmer has mentioned.

These descriptions briefly give the body-constitutional side of the typology of Kretschmer. We have already indicated a few of the relations between the physical constitutions of Kretschmer and W. Jaensch such as the eyes and skin. In later chapters more and more relations will in the course of our expositions be shown. This does not only apply to the types of Jaensch, but also to the endocrine types of Berman, Pende, Breitmann, etc. ; the bio-types of Ewald, Mathes, Weininger, Huter, etc. ; the common anthropological racial types. We do not by any means contemplate a treatment of all these elaborate typologies ; but we are strongly of the opinion that the Kretschmer-types, with which we deal here primarily, are by no means unique. It becomes more and more evident that with further accumulation of results it will be possible in the near future to reduce all these typologies to the same simple formula of biological principles. Accordingly, while dealing with the Kretschmer types it is both attractive and necessary to compare them with aspects of the other types. Also, where we are attempting to reach sharper differentiations

in the types both on the physical and mental sides, the
other typologies sometimes are of considerable assistance.

15. *Races*

The anthropological races are also described by
measurements and in terms of a similar kind as that of
Kretschmer's types. A vast amount of work has been
done by anthropologists on racial characteristics and
it will be instructive from the physical side briefly to
compare here some of these characteristics with those
of Kretschmer's types as outlined in this chapter. To
me it seems to be fairly obvious—and it has already been
stated by authorities [1]—that there are intimate relationships between the leptosome constitution and the Nordic
race, the pyknic constitution and the Alpine race, the
athletic constitution and the Dinaric race of Europe.
It is a foolish issue to decide whether Kretschmer merely
dealt with different races or whether anthropologists
described Kretschmer's types, especially at the present
state of racial admixture. One thing seems certain, and
that is that a large percentage of the Nordics are athletic
leptosomes, of the Alpinics are pyknics, and of the
Dinarics are athletics. Let us mention a few of the
physical characteristics of each which seem to prove this :—

Nordics and leptosomes : Tall and slender bodies ;
length of legs and arms ; receding forehead ; long, narrow
nose with tip drawn downwards ; thin lips (such
characteristics as the strong beard of the Nordics indicates
that there are also important differences).

---

[1] Gunther, *Rassenkunde*, 1929, p. 169. It is, however, refuted, e.g.
by Henckel, who shows that in territories predominantly inherited
by one or other of these races all the constitution types are found.
The question whether races are really only constitution types can, as
Gunther points out, hardly be decided. Even if this were proved to
be the case, that would only show that the different environments to
which these races after their common origin were subjected, acted
selectively to produce the divergence. But the actual explanation must
even then be found in physiological conditions eventually. Refer also,
L. Polen, *Archiv. f. d. Ges. Psychologie*, Bd. 66, pp. 1–116. The types
of Kretschmer are also found in the S.A. Bantu—physically as well as
temperamentally (vide Fig. 48).

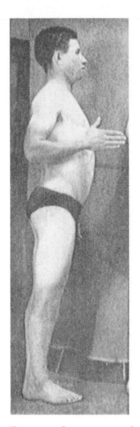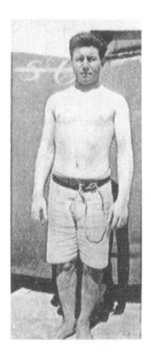

FIG. 24. Same person, but right was taken eight months after left; in meantime boy had developed a pasty fat layer.

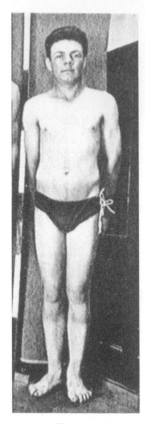

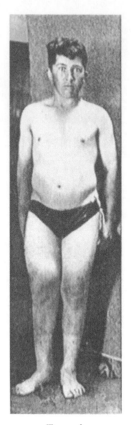

FIG. 25.   FIG. 26.

[face p 61

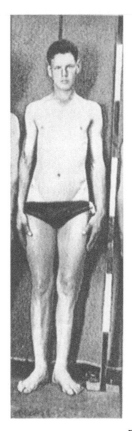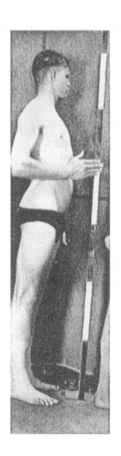

FIG. 27.

[face p. 60

Athletics and Dinarics : Remarkable tallness ; steep back of head ; " high head " ; prominent nose with high bridge ; characteristic form of the lower jaw ; coarse features throughout ; large ears (the athletics of our material, however, show many Nordic characteristics as well).

Pyknics and Alpinics : Small height ; thick-set, compact ; broad head, short thick neck ; short legs ; fat accumulation on neck and trunk ; full-moon face ; prominent dome-shaped forehead ; small to medium nose with bridge sometimes bent inwards.

On the mental side there are also many interesting points of correspondence. We shall, in footnotes, refer to some of these similarities as we continue. Here we may perhaps mention some interesting facts on the mental side as found by the Jaensch school.[1] E. R. Jaensch indicates that in experimental research on school children, the French proved to belong to the B-type (K's cyclotype) much more frequently than the Germans of Marburg. Also, W. Jaensch states that the B-type is frequently connected with dark hair and a dark iris, the T-type with fair hair, etc. W. Jaensch admits frankly that the T-type has relations with the Nordic race.

[1] E. R. Jaensch, " Zur differentiellen Volkerpsychologie," 8th *Kongress f. Expt. Psych.*, Leipzig, 1923 ; W. Jaensch, *Grundzüge*, pp. 108, 146, 147, 163.

CHAPTER IV

The Mental Side of the Schizo-Type

16. *The Schizo-personality* [1]

In his classical work, *Physique and Character*, Kretschmer has, with unparalleled vividness, richness and naturalness of metaphor, described the two great temperament complexes or temperament systems : the one ranges from the normal healthy Schizothyme, over the borderline cases or psychopaths, viz. Schizoids, to the fully insane Schizophrenes. The other begins with the normal healthy Cyclothyme, over the borderline cases of Cycloids, to the insane Manic-depressives or Circulars. He conceives the definitely insane as a strong caricature of the same fundamental temperamental proportions that we find in normal life. His theory begins with the investigation of pre-and post-psychotic patients and their nearest blood relatives and finally is applied to healthy normals, historical persons in science, art, politics, etc.[2] He tries to bring the members of each of the two great temperament types, both normal and abnormal, into one large picture. Thus we get the two large personality pictures : the Schizo's and the Cyclo's. The former shows a biological affinity to the Leptosomic, Athletic and Dysplastic contitution type, while the latter has a biological affinity to the Pyknic constitution type.[3]

---

[1] We presuppose acquaintance on the part of the reader with the main work of Kretschmer at least. Even those who cannot agree with many of the basic principles of Kretschmer's theory have admitted his unparalleled genius in the exposition of these personality-types, e.g. Schneider, *Psychologie der Schizo-phrenen*, p. 211.

[2] Vide also Kretschmer. *The Psychology of Men of Genius.*

[3] The reader must bear with me for the apparently indiscriminate use of such terms as " personality ", " temperament ", " constitution ", " character ", etc. I intentionally refrain from giving definitions at the beginning, because terms such as " psychæsthetic proportions ", " psycho-motility ", " volitional attitude ", " perseveration ", will be

With regard to the gradual transitions from the healthy Cyclothyme through the Cycloid to the definitely insane Circular, most of the foremost authorities in Psychiatry, such as Bumke, Bleuler, Thalbitzer, McDougall,[1] etc., are in agreement. But many authorities in psychiatry disagree with Kretschmer's theory that Schizophrenia is merely a hyper-accentuation, a caricature of the normal Schizothyme personality proportions (*vide* Bumke, C. Schneider, Willmanns, Gruhle, Lange, etc.).[2] Some of these, notably Bumke, conceive Schizoids, i.e. border-line cases, to be normal personalities with disease " tones " or modifications just like a white race with coloured influences, but any connections between the normal Schizothyme and the disease Schizophrenia they reject. On the other hand, nearly all authorities from Kraepelin to those of the present day have found a large percentage of " peculiars ", " eccentrics ", " timid, shy sensitives ", " cold egotists ", idealists ", and " dreamers ", amongst the blood relatives of Schizophrenes, and also in the pre-psychotic personalities of Schizophrenes. The central characteristic of all these personalities is the " defective capacity to adapt (Einfügung) sincerely, frankly and easily to the social environment ".[3] Moreover, C. Schneider, an opponent of Kretschmer's doctrines, after consideration of all modern investigations, states that the pre-psychotic characteristics mentioned are retained in the typical Schizophrenic social behaviour, i.e. the eccentricity acts pathoplastically; and the typical pre-psychotic personality traits, such as sensitive reserve, determine

used in my definitions. These latter terms are only explained in the sequel as they come, and, being somewhat individual and uncommon terms, cannot be used to explain the former. It would be very much like defining the known in terms of the unknown, because most readers know more or less what we mean by temperament, etc., but not so clearly what we mean by " psychæsthetic proportions ".

[1] O. Bumke, *Lehrbuch der Geisteskrankheiten*, München, 1929, pp. 209, 327. Bleuler, *Psychiatrie*, 1929 ; Thalbitzer, *Emotion and Insanity*, London, 1926 ; McDougall, *Outline of Abnormal Psychology*, London, 1926.

[2] Bumke, *op. cit.*, pp. 209, 680 ; C. Schneider, *Psychologie der Schizophrenen*, 1930, p. 225.

[3] C. Schneider, *op. cit.*, p. 218.

or constitute some of the essential features of Schizophrenic mind. We are not in a position to discuss the advisability of conceiving the Schizophrenic mind as an extreme caricature of the normal Schizothyme mind. Even if later psychiatric research shows this to be improbable, the " Schizothyme temperament ", i.e. the temperament prevalent in pre-psychotic persons and their blood relatives, remains a valuable working hypothesis.[1]

Kretschmer gives the essential features of the Schizothyme temperament in this order of frequency :—

(1) Unsociable, quiet, reserved, serious-minded, eccentric.
(2) Timid, shy, with fine feelings, sensitive, nervous, excitable, fond of nature and books.
(3) Pliable, kindly, honest, indifferent, dull-witted, silent.

He sub-divides them into the following sub-types [2] :—

Hyperæsthetics : Nervous excitables, tender introverts, idealists.
Medium Schizothymes : Cool energetics, systematic consequents, composed aristocrats.
Anæsthetics : Cold nervous, distorted eccentrics, indolents, affectively lame, dull-witted loafers.

These characteristics, accordingly, we should find in leptosomes, athletes and dysplastics. It is at once obvious that on the psychical as well as on the physical side we are dealing with very broad, heterogeneous groups, and

---

[1] Even if Schizophrenia as a mental disease has no inherent relations to Schizothymia, the value of psychopathology in this problem remains unshaken. It was only possible to isolate this type of personality in clinical experience with Schizophrenes because : either the Schizothymic temperament is more pronounced in pre-psychotic persons and their blood relations, or because in the Schizophrene group the pyknics are not present (they are not prone to Schizophrenia but to manic-depression), so that the Schizothyme mind is only the normal mind minus the Cyclothyme components (Bumke's idea), or the disease, Schizophrenia, has an affinity for certain body-types, just as the normal Schizothyme temperament has an affinity for the same body-types, without there being any immediate connection between Schizophrenia and the Schizothyme temperament. From C. Schneider's long drawn out and ingenious criticisms of Kretschmer's " Schizothyme " theory, however, one gets the impression that what they really differ about is the name. If " Sonderlinge " (peculiars, eccentrics) be substituted for " Schizo-thyme, -id ", they would have been more or less reconciled.

[2] Kretschmer, *Medizinische Psychologie*, Leipzig, 1930, p. 155.

that very much of the practical value of the Schizothyme type is lost because of the loose correlations with various physique types. Subsequent researches on the Schizothyme physique types, however, have made the following relations probable [1] :—

(1) The leptosome is really the true Schizo-physique, because leptosomes more than any other types are prone to Schizophrenia.

(2) The athletic is more frequently connected with the " epileptoid " character.

(3) Dysplastics form the bulk of the " epileptic " characters.

17 *Differences between Leptosomes and Athletics*

We saw that on the physique side there are important similarities between leptosomes and athletics. But there are also such striking differences between these two types on the physique side that, if the temperament and the physique are at all narrowly connected, we must expect to find correspondingly strong differences between the temperaments of these two types. Such differences have, as we stated in the previous paragraph, been found both on psychopathological and experimental evidence. Athletics and dysplastics certainly have intimate connections with the Schizothyme group. But Kretschmer [2] and his followers have found statistically, and he has expressed this unequivocally, that : " The leptosomes appear as the predominating type of the Schizo-group." According to Peritz,[3] Berman, etc., the endocrine personalities, viz. the tetanoid and status thymico lymphaticus, who are susceptible to Schizophrenia, are undoubtedly of the leptosomic bodybuild and not so much

[1] We admit that this statement requires a substantial confirmation. In the sequel we shall, in the proper order, adduce all the results and considerations, which we know of, to substantiate these important statements.

[2] Kretschmer, *Medizinische Psychologie*, 4th ed., Leipzig, 1930, p. 158.

[3] Peritz, *Einführung in die Klinik der Inneren Sekretion*, Berlin, pp. 165, 184, 245, 250.

athletic.   Ewald,[1] reviewing the present state of the body-temperament theories, states that Kretschmer is certainly near the truth when he attempts closer correlations in the following manner : leptosomic and asthenic physique types tend to affective crampedness (Affektverkrämpfung), love abstract thinking, are angular and unfree in their movements, tend to sexual conflicts (intersexual type of Mathes).   Ewald also mentions that athletics and dysplastics often show explosive affectivity, formerly called epileptoid.   The statistical studies of Kretschmer and his followers on clinical material support these views that leptosomes predominate in pure Schizophrenia and athletics and dysplastics in the epileptic syndrome.[2]   In 175 Schizophrenes Kretschmer found 81 leptosomes (= 46 per cent), and only 31 athletics (= 18 per cent) and 34 dysplastics (= 19 per cent).   In epilepsy (700 cases) intensive investigations showed the relative insignificant percentage of leptosomes ($\pm$ 12 per cent) as compared with Athletics ($\pm$ 32 per cent) and dysplastics ($\pm$ 45 per cent).   Langfeldt in an extended investigation found leptosomes predominantly amongst catatonics with significant other qualities, such as a very low basal metabolism and soft testes.   Athletics on the other hand, he found to be more common in hebephrenias.   They showed a normal basal metabolism and hard testes.   He also believed to have shown differences in sympathetico- and vagotonic in these subdivisions of Schizophrenia.[3]   Wexberg [4] indicates that leptosomes predominate in psycho-reactive depressions (he even speaks of Schizoid depressions), but that athletics are more seldom among these anxious and self-insufficient feeling persons.   Wexberg also quotes an investigation of Professor Lange, who found only one pyknic and 9 asthenics

[1] Professor G. Ewald, *Die Körperliche Grundlagen des Charakters*, Leipzig, 1928.
[2] *Physique and Character*, p. 35 ; Kreyenberg, *Körperbau, Epilepsie und Charakter*, p. 508.   He worked under the personal guidance of Kretschmer.   Similar results were obtained by Delbrück, v. Rohden, Mauz, Grundler, Kleist, etc.
[3] *D. Ztschft. f. Nervenheilkunde* 1927, Bd. 97, p. 133.
[4] E. Wexberg, *Ztschft. f. d. Ges. Neur. und Psychiatrie*, Bd. 112, p. 549.

(leptosomes), but no athletics, amongst 11 cases of psychogenic depression.

In a recent article,[1] Kretschmer has acknowledged the connections between athletics and dysplastics on the one hand, and the epileptoid character qualities on the other.

On the experimental psychological side, a follower of Kretschmer, Enke,[2] has also established many important differences between athletics and leptosomes : both types are much more subject to persistent cramped attentive attitudes (intentions), and to perseveration generally, than the pyknic type, but leptosomes were much more so than athletics. The same can be said of the ability to do different tasks simultaneously. In handwriting Enke found that athletics differ strongly from leptosomes in the pressure on the nib, angularity of writing, etc. (vide Fig. 34).[3] These differences in handwriting are symptomatic of differences in temperament (Klages, Saudek). A very important fact is that according to our own and Enke's experimental finding, leptosomes are the best in small, delicate hand movements, while pyknics come second, and athletics are the worst. This is found to be so in spite of the fact that leptosomes are more shaky, due to " strong inner tensions " (excitement). Athletics often handled " the lever-arms very clumsily " and corrected their drawings by " making use of excessive force ". Throughout Enke's descriptions the impression is created that the leptosomes are more accurate, more nervously anxious to excel and more wary against pitfalls than the athletics. In a test where hesitations depended on suspicion, on the tendency to safeguarding, " assurances " in Adler's sense, reserve and care of the subjects, such hesitations were found

---

[1] *Deutsche Jur. Zeit.*, 31, p. 785.

[2] Enke, " Die Psychomotorik der Konstitutionstypen," *Ztschft. f. Ang. Psych.*, Bd. 36, pp. 254, 257, 261, 277, 283. Kretschmer, *Med. Psych.*, p. 158.

[3] This example is from our own investigations in connection with the handwriting of types. Mr. R. E. Lighton, of our institute, will shortly publish the results of these investigations.

in 25 per cent of the pyknics, 61 per cent of the athletics, and 80 per cent of the leptosomes.

These facts and considerations clearly indicate that attempts are being made to arrive at a differentiation between the leptosomes and the athletics on psycho-pathological and experimental psychological grounds. The results seem to be that the leptosomes form the typical Schizo-type, while the athletics must be considered in the light of the epileptoid studies and according to Delbrück's [1] proportion of " Driven-Bound ".

Also, in his individual analyses of temperaments in his earlier works, Kretschmer frequently indicates that the bulk of his Schizo-group who have the " sensitive affectively lame " temperaments, also have long, slender bodies, e.g. such phrases as " Hölderlin type," " mimosa natures," " hyperæsthetics of but little strength, little resistance and weakly impulsed," " hot-house-like, blooming of an inner world," are found together with sexual immaturity, mother-fixation, social timidity, and above all, in descriptions of long, lean bodies, thin noses long thin hands. This unmistakably indicates the leptosome and especially the more asthenic bodybuild in conjunction with such temperaments.[2]

Apart from the results in Kretschmer s own institute and the psychopathological evidence, other investigators in more practical fields have found significant differences between leptosomes and athletics. Pfahler [3] believes that in art the leptosomes may be more inclined to the group of romantics (i.e. sensitive, tender, feminine, retiring

---

[1] Delbrück, *Archiv. f. Psych. und Nervenkrankheiten*, Bd. 82, 1928, p. 708.

[2] It is true that Kretschmer also describes the cold insensitive types in " long, lean frames " ; but he expressly states that, " the sensitive-affectively lame, in its whole range from the timid, weakly, emoted schizoid imbecile up to the highly differentiated Hölderlin natures are perhaps the most important schizoid type of temperament ; at any rate one of the most frequent pre-psychotic foundations." The cold, insensitive types which Kretschmer describes are mostly " post-psychotic " personalities, and in this mixing of the post-psychotic traits, i.e. disease traits, with normal pre-psychotic traits lies Kretschmer's great weakness (C. Schneider, K. Schneider, Jaspers, Bumke, Wilmanns).

[3] Pfahler, *System der Typenlehren*, Leipzig, 1929, p. 183.

individuals) and the elegiacs, while athletics may represent the pathetics (more strongly flavoured, impulsive and active natures) and satirics. Lenz [1] has found, as we shall see in the sequel, great differences between the leptosomic and athletic criminal. The same can be said of studies on criminals by Professor Böhmer.[2]

These differences between leptosomes and athletics, etc., on the psychical side are very important from a theoretical and practical point of view. Wahle [3] has tried to some extent to ridicule the body-temperament theory of Kretschmer by pointing out that extremely powerful, robust body-builds, fall into the same temperament-group with the exact opposite body-build of the weakly and tender.[4] Also, as long as we cannot differentiate on the psychical side between leptosomes and athletics, very little practical value, e.g. in delinquency, can be derived from the typology.

Even if the main difference between the athletic and leptosomic personality is in the asthenic-sthenic form of experiencing and reaction—a quality in close reciprocal relations with body strength—this would, as we shall indicate, make a remarkable difference in delinquency.

18 *Leptosome personality and delinquency : Asthenic experiencing*

(a) *General orientations about the asthenic experiencing of leptosomes.*

" Our psychical relation to the external world is a play of forces in which we alternately have on the one hand, the consciousness of superiority, of joyful power, of control and action ; on the other, the consciousness of inferiority, of discouraged submission, of defeat and

---

[1] A. Lenz, *Grundriss der Kriminalbiologie.*
[2] K. Bohmer, *Monatschrift f. Kriminalpsychologie*, Heidelberg, 1928, pp. 193–209.
[3] Quoted by Pfahler, *op. cit.*, p. 182.
[4] The differences between the leptosomes and athletics will also become more evident in chapter IX where the biophysiological bases of the types are discussed.

shame." [1] Some human beings are more disposed to the former, the sthenic, form of experiencing and attitude towards the outside world ; others, again, are more disposed to the latter, the asthenic, form of experiencing and attitude towards the external world. These sthenic-asthenic antipoles of psychical behaviour have been worked out elaborately by Ewald [2] in his scheme of characters. But as far as I am aware, the purely psychical polarity of sthenic-asthenic has not been definitely co-ordinated with physique types. In fact, K. Schneider warns against the simple predication of asthenic temperamental qualities to the asthenic physical habitus.

We have found, however, and shall indicate this fully in the sequel, that the more one moves away from athletic mixtures towards the pure leptosome and the asthenic bodybuild, the more frequently does one also meet with asthenic temperamental qualities. Asthenic temperamental qualities, or asthenic attitude, form of experience and reaction, are here to be understood as the opposite of sthenic qualities in the sense of Kretschmer's definition given above, or according to the scheme of Ewald. Such asthenic qualities are as follows : Weak self-confidence, sense of insecurity, timidity, shyness, hesitation, reserve, inhibitions, etc. On the other hand, as we move from the asthenic physique through the pure leptosome towards the athletic leptosome and the leptosomic athletic physiques, the attitude towards life and the environment becomes more and more sthenic. We find an increase of the following sthenic qualities (in the above sense) :—Love of responsibility, leadership qualities, strong and persistent energy physically as well as psychically, boastfulness, self-confidence, unyielding obstinacy, intractability, active jealousy, sarcasm, sportsmanship, love of adventure, active ambition, sulkiness, systematic mistrust, etc.

[1] *Med. Psych.*, p. 194.
[2] Ewald, *Temperament und Charakter*, Berlin, 1924, and also Hoffmann, *Aufbau der Persönlichkeit*, p. 42. Lenz, *Kriminalbiologie*, p. 168, also quotes Jung to show that psychoasthenia is the prevalent disease of introverts.

Where in the sequel we shall attempt to establish this relation between asthenic-sthenic mental qualities on the one hand and leptosomic (including asthenic) and athletic physical habitus on the other hand, the terms asthenic temperament and experiencing must not be confused with the asthenic habitus. The two applications of " asthenic "—once to a type of mental behaviour and again to a particular somatic condition—must be clearly distinguished.

The leptosome described by Kretschmer is nearer the asthenic physique as some later writers, e.g. van der Velde,[1] have interpreted it. In fact, in his original works Kretschmer used the term asthenic for the general form (now termed leptosome) as well as for the extreme weakly variant (now termed asthenic). It is important to note this, because the type which is so prone to schizophrenia and which we are here discussing as leptosome, is usually comparatively weakly built or, more definitely, is nothing more or less than that described in paragraph 9. This long, lean type with thin muscles, etc., is the same type as that described by Peritz in connection with tetanoid, by Eppinger and Hess as vagotonic. It has intimate biological connections with the status thymico lymphaticus which is already an early puberty extreme. These types are taken to be asthenically inclined psychically by Peritz and others. We also find that the class of Schizothyme temperaments most frequent in Kretschmer's pre-psychotic personalities, viz. the " sensitive, affectively lame ",[2] is made up mainly of asthenic, psychical qualities. He states definitely that the passionate-insensitive or brutal variants of the Schizoid group are usually post-psychotics,

---

[1] Th. v. d. Velde, *De Bestryding der Echtelyken Afkeer*, Leiden, 1927.

[2] *Physique and Character*, p. 168, " The type of the sensitive-affectively lame . . . the most important schizoid type of temperament, at any rate one of the most frequent pre-psychotic foundations and starting points." Indeed, most of Kretschmer's characterization of the Schizoid gives this impression. The insensitive brutal type is usually a post-psychotic wreck (p. 169) with many connections with certain brain traumatic and epileptic syndromes (p. 170). Also, vide Peritz, *Innere Sekretion*, 245, 250.

i.e. persons whose more delicate super personality structures have been devastated by a Schizophrenia attack.   He also mentions that the passionate-insensitive outbursts have many connections with certain brain-traumatic and epileptic syndromes.[1]   These syndromes we shall later bring into relation with degenerate athletics.   Our contention is, therefore, that the leptosomes, as described by Kretschmer, and more particularly the asthenically built leptosomes, are inclined towards the asthenic form of experiencing.   This we believe to be supported by Kretschmer's own findings because the most common form of Schizoid according to Kretschmer, is the timid one, and the most common physique in the Schizoid group is the leptosome (or asthenic) physique. We may, therefore, expect a fair correlation between timidity and leptosomy. If we go more into details it is not difficult to prove that asthenic characteristics figure largely in Kretschmer's descriptions of the Schizothyme temperament, and also in the Schizoid pre-psychotic temperament.   Compare such qualities as mother-fixation, fear with tears of a tyrant father, sexual hesitancy and timid excitement in relations with girls, fear of rough school games, submission to teasing by school-fellows, excitable timid nervousness, homesickness in a boy of 17, fear at the sight of blood, tender hyper-æsthetics, of but little strength, little resistance and weakly impulsed, hothouselike blooming inwards to escape the harsh contacts with the external world.   Such characteristics, which are the most prevalent in Schizothymes, demonstrate indubitably that the leptosome is largely asthenic temperamentally.[2]   The sensitivity is also largely due to such asthenic qualities with a sthenic " strain or antipole ",[3] firmly rooted in the asthenic framework.

[1] *Physique and Character*, pp. 169 and 170.
[2] W. Jaensch in characterizing the T-type, which corresponds to Kretschmer's Schizoid, quotes Professor Kroh : " The typical tetanoid is often restless, anxious, insecure, and suspicious " (*Grundzuge*, p. 126).
[3] Kretschmer, *Med. Psych.*, p. 199.   Kretschmer is an acknowledged authority on the genesis and intrinsic nature of Sensitive Paranoia which he explains in this way as an asthenic-sthenic function.

Idealistic, erotic, or egoconscious ambition usually provides such a strain or antipole. The asthenic temperamental characteristics and the sensitivity of the leptosome are inextricably interwoven with his sexual peculiarities or anomalies, his autism or defective social congenial adaptations, his love of nature and solitude, his idealism and abstract thinking. The more we analyse all these intrinsic qualities of the leptosome group of Schizothymes, the more clearly it dawns upon us that these qualities are only different aspects of the same fundamental bio-psychological complex. As we shall see in later chapters, too, we simply cannot explain the negative, self-insufficient, vulnerable, shrinking and blooming inwards attitude of the leptosome as due to the experiences of continuous defeats in all fields of natural adaptation. We know, for instance, that masculinity, aggressiveness, anger, muscularity, physical strength and endurance have, also in the animal world, intimate connections with the adrenal cortex, the prepituitary and the male interstitial glands and their neural controls.[1] The aggressiveness or submissiveness is therefore not a result of experience only, but is determined neuroglandularly. The same applies to feminine coyness, submissiveness to the male, tenderhearted nervousness, lack of sexual aggressiveness. These feminine characteristics are very similar to many of the leptosomic characteristics and, as we shall see later on, there is much of " intersexuality " in the leptosomic physical constitution.[2] We also know at the present day that in the first stages of puberty we

---

[1] Berman, *Glands Regulating Personality*, New York, 1928, pp. 72, 188, 196, 243, also Pende, *Konstitution und Inneren Sekretion*, Messina, 1924, pp. 12, 22, 24, 38.

[2] Mathes, the eminent authority on female constitutional types, *Handbuch der Frauenheilkunde*, Bd. 3, Vienna, takes the leptosome as an intersexual type. The intersexuality of the leptosome is also evident from the following : Frequent homosexuality ; close somatic relationship with the Status Thymicus (Pende, p. 39 ; Berman, pp. 251, 266), where male sex glands are inhibited ; somatic and psychic similarities with Eunuchoidism ; correspondences with early puberty phase when sexuality is still weakly differentiated. Cf. also, Ewald, *op. cit.*, p. 51, and Peritz, *op. cit.*

have a similar asthenic, retreating, hypersensitive, introvertive phase termed the "negation-period" by Charlotte Bühler.[1] This attitude towards life is definitely and largely determined by physiological causes, i.e. is not purely an acquired attitude produced by experiences of a harsh world. This genetic phase of the human personality has, as we shall see all along, on the physical, sexual, and temperamental sides, exceedingly intimate correspondence with the leptosome constitution and can therefore serve such purposes of comparison adequately. In many cases of an asthenic attitude towards the outside world, however, experience and constitutional dispositions work together to produce the temperamental state. This may give some explanation of sometimes athletics are sometimes hypochondriacal, weakly impulsed and retreative. But, as we shall see further on, one must be very careful in diagnosing individuals as asthenic temperamentally in the athletic type, because they may sham weakness to escape penal servitude. Athletics are very unemotional and therefore may be inactive without the subjective feeling of inferiority or weakness ; and also dysplastic constitutional features may change the constitutional reactive tendencies of athletics considerably. Numerous considerations in following chapters will give more support to our contention that the more we move to the physical asthenic build the more childlike, self-insufficient, feministic, submissive, and lacking in manly aggressiveness they become : towards the athletic muscular side, the more the bold, aggressively active and real masculine tendencies increase. The biological implications are, as we shall see, extremely interesting and significant for our biological bases of the typological differences. This asthenic temperament is seen very strikingly in the causes and nature of the delinquency of leptosomes.

---

[1] Throughout this work we shall endeavour to show very intimate correspondences between the leptosome constitution and the early pubertial phase as described by Professor Ch. Bühler, *Das Seelenleben des Jugendlichen*, Jena, 1927, and Professor Ed. Spranger, *Psychologie des Jugendalters*, Leipzig, 1926.

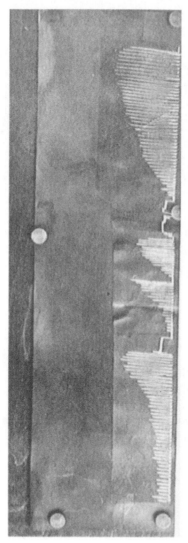

[face p. 74

FIG. 28.   Change of form of ergogram with successive performances; 30 seconds rest between each and a decrease in weight from 5 kg. to 4, 3, 2 kgr. resp., starting from the right.

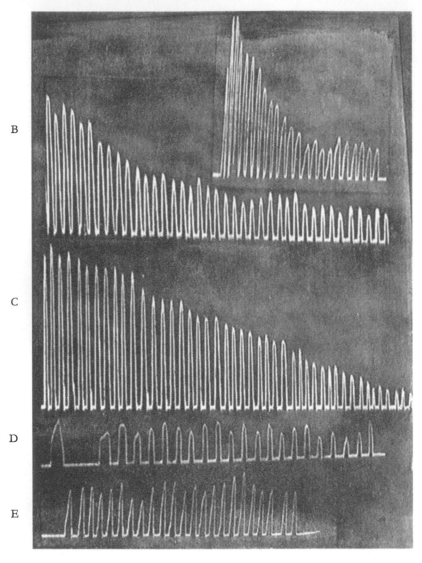

FIG. 29.   A, Fatigued muscle.   B, Concave ergogram.   C, Triangle form.
D and E, Formless (infantile).

[face p. 75

(b) Physical inactivity.

Skawran [1] has demonstrated that his concave ergogram type is found mainly in the more asthenically built leptosomes and infantilistic physique types. In the delinquent material, from which he has also largely drawn, this was very striking. The following cases drew extremely concave ergograms (vide Fig. 29 b).

Case 3.—Age 16. Convicted for housebreaking and theft. Broke into private house of a woman during morning hours by climbing through window when he knew that occupant was out. Stole 15s. and a mounted 5s. piece. Told his mother that he had obtained money at school. First offence was theft of 12s. from a Native hut when occupants were away.[2] Conduct in reformatory colourless, slow, but exemplary. Offences in reformatory : Filthy, immoral talk ; leaving bed without permission ; assisting other boys to escape—tried to abscond himself, but was captured ; smoking ; neglect of work ; negligence to report irons of bed to be loose. He was released on good conduct to a farmer. Absconded from this farm because he did not like to work ; proved very lazy, weakly, and incapable at farm work. General characterizations : Weak ambition, very timid, and no energy. In march, always listless plodder at end of the rank. Dull-witted, placid, though good-natured, and if addressed sympathetically gives a friendly, shy smile. Subaltern, suggestible, slow. Sniffs his nose feebly—too timid to sniff forcibly. His physique is asthenic leptosome (vide Fig. 14 right).

Case 4.—Age 17. Convicted five times of stock theft (fowls) and once of theft of wood from forest and coal from coalyard. Father diseased, mother very poor and backward. Offences in reformatory, nil. Parasitic, weakling, timid, longboned, placid, dull-witted type. My observations were : placid, mummy face. Unable to appreciate any jokes made during tests ; dissatisfied, lame expression. His energy weak—not only on account of weak muscles, but cramped affectivity. Evil-smelling breath, sores on lips and legs. Mouth hanging open. Timidly peeped at me

---

[1] Skawran, *Typology of Ergograms*.
[2] I have just received information (fourteen months after the above investigation) that this boy, who had since been released on good conduct, has again stolen money, etc., from a Native hut, and therefore been recommitted to the reformatory.

sideways. Unsociable, no interest in boys' games or conversation. Lies in sun on edge of football ground. Tries his best in tests. Physically a fairly pure (perhaps slightly asthenic) leptosome.

These are extreme cases where the lack of initiative and real social activity seems to be the main and uncomplicated cause of their delinquency. They are real asthenic, passive parasites who have to steal in a cowardly, petty manner to find a living. Their ergograms are extreme " defatigation curves " (vide Fig. 29 b) which have been shown by Skawran to correspond to the ergogram of a fatigued person.[1] We may therefore assume as proved by experiment, observations, and nature of delinquency that this type of leptosome lacks true activity. We have found such weak energy in a very large percentage of leptosomes in the reformatory. In many cases, as we shall see, the lack of energy was complicated by other qualities, such as calculativeness, autism, introversion, compensations, sexual problems, etc. It is rather surprising to find this large proportion of weakly-impulsed leptosomes in view of the fact that Skawran shows the normal leptosome to have a fair tenacity in life and in his experiments. This tenacity depends largely on their attempts to vindicate their sensitive (self-insufficient) and subtly developed ego-consciousness.[2] But Skawran mentions also in his work that the simple triangular ergogram (not the concave form) drawn by these tenacious leptosomes come from the " well developed leptosomes " with frequent athletic admixture (vide Fig. 29 c). The concave fatigue curves mostly derive from infantilistic

[1] Skawran found that this concave type of curve corresponded closely to that of a fatigued muscle and innervation system. He made the person rest for 30 seconds after he had pulled the first time to exhaustion, and then continue to pull with a weight of 4 kgrs. instead of 5 kgrs.—the original weight. After the second exhaustion, again 30 seconds rest, and the weight to be pulled further diminished by 1 kgr., and so on. In this way, he proved that all persons eventually showed a concave ergogram as they became more depleted physically (vide Fig. 28).

[2] Numerous investigations have led to a strong emphasis on this aspect of the leptosomic personality. It is a form of compensation, a sensitive development on the basis of an asthenic form of experiencing with a sthenic antipole or sting. Cf. Skawran, *op. cit.* ; Enke, *op. cit.*, pp. 251, 255, 258 ; Kretschmer ; W. Jaensch, *op. cit.*

and weakly, thinly built leptosomes and persons generally lacking both in good muscles and attitude-dispositions to overcome the fatigue. The weakly impulsed, inactive leptosome bulks so largely in the delinquent material, exactly because this inactivity is such a formidable cause of his delinquency.

(c) Submission to evil influences.

Many of the asthenic temperaments are naturally, as a result of passive self-insufficiency feelings towards more heroic natures, very susceptible to influences. They are unable to resist the self-confident semi-hypnotic domination, especially of the robust mixtures of pyknics and athletics ; moreover, they feel safer and covered by the bold initiative and leadership of these types.[1] We need not labour this characteristic. The following cases speak for themselves :—

> *Case 5.*—Age 18. With two other juveniles older than himself, and two adults, one of whom was his brother, he was convicted of many store-breaks, involving several hundred pounds worth of goods stolen, over a lengthy period. His brother (short and well-built) told him that if he went with the gang he would receive many fine clothes. He was directly willing to go, but states definitely that he was too afraid to go alone, and would never have done anything without his brother's protection and persuasion. When charged by the detectives, he immediately confessed everything. My observations of the boy were : Smiled shyly but good-naturedly ; inactive ; weak initiative. Record shows that he changed work several times, in some cases only because he had to rise too early or had to collect money from unwilling debtors of his employer. Unemployed for more than a year at time of arrest. Is a subaltern quiet type, the lame suggestible leptosome, unable to overcome the influence of others under whose protection he stole at places where they could not be easily detected. In his letters, longs for home ; asks his people not to forget him.

We have many such cases, where leptosomes of the asthenic kind are used or influenced by more robust

---

[1] The tendency to seek protection, help, and understanding from older and stronger persons is also mentioned by Ch. Bühler as a typical early puberty characteristic, *op. cit.*, pp. 64, 77, 156.

persons to accompany them. The conditions take on a slightly different colour when such inferior-feeling leptosomes or eunuchoid-inclined persons are used by others in evil practices or persuaded to take the blame on themselves. Such instances we encountered in a few cases of sodomy and in one case such a lame wretch with a low mentality was apparently used by his own father to bear the blame of the father's stock theft.

> *Case* 6.—Age 18. Stole watch, fountain pen, pocket book, etc., from an open portmanteau in a railway caboose, belonging to a former employer. The caboose was unattended and the boy knew where and how these things were kept. No offences in reformatory, but without energy and backbone. Warden says he is a real " mother's child ". " Mammie " like a little child in his letters. Somewhat sly attitude in testroom. No exertion on football field. Extreme lack of self-confidence and manly self-assertion. Said he had less brains than another boy examined with him when I remarked that his head measurements exceeded that of the other boy. He was used for sodomy by the other boys, and afterwards cried bitterly about it—stating that he had done such a great sin. His body-type is very interesting (Fig. 14 lft). Very long legs (94 cm.), certainly something of an elongated eunuchoid (Hochwuchs) ; upper spine bent forwards ; head rather low between shoulders ; feministic facial skin and features, well-rounded pelvical contour makes a strong feminine impression. The hypo-plastic chin, shortened-egg-form frontal view of face and physical features generally are those of the leptosome type.

This case also shows the very intimate correspondence physically and psychically of the " intersexual " type with the leptosome type, the sly, self-insecure, submissive attitude these types have in common.[1] We have another example where subjection to homosexual practices of other boys is found together with a pure leptosome physique and a typical leptosome delinquency. For general purposes of exposition of the leptosome temperament, this case may accordingly be analysed in detail :—

[1] Berman, *Glands Regulating Personality*, p. 261 ; Kretschmer, *Med. Psychologie*, p. 62 ; Peritz, *Innere Sekretion*, p. 249 ; Ebbecke, *X Kongress f. Expt. Psych.*, Bonn, 1927 ; Lenz, *Grundriss*, p. 115.

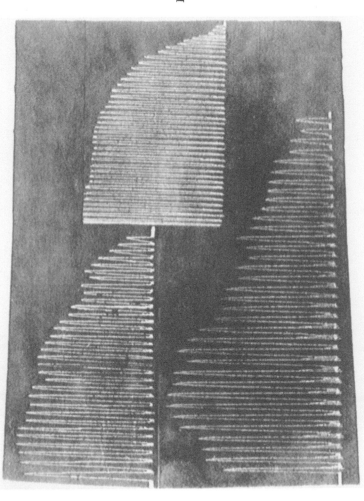

Fig. 30. A, Convex ergogram. B, Rectangle form. C, Mixed convex.

[face p. 78

Case 7.—Age 16. Forgery and uttering. In name of a farmer he knew to be addicted to drink, he wrote letters for a native to buy brandy at a bottle store. He received 2*s*. 6*d*. three times and 1*s*. once in payment of several such notes. The native was known to the family on the farm for years, and afterwards worked in a garage in town as driver of a motor lorry. The boy boarded in the village school hostel (Std. VII) and only went home during week-ends. The native worried him daily for notes with which to buy brandy; sobbed, begged, bribed, and afterwards threatened the boy. One day the native told the boy that he would take him to the farm on the motor lorry he drove, if the boy would write such a note for him. The boy being very fond of his home-life and the farm, could no longer withstand bribes and threats, and eventually acceded. After some days the native came again and threatened to report the first note if the boy did not write another one for him. This went on for months with begging and bribing on the one side, and threats on the other, until the native was arrested for drunkenness. The boy immediately confessed.

Our observations : A real leptosome physique, delicately boned and very thin muscles, somewhat girlish complexion, short-egg-face. Temperamentally the quiet, timid, lover of nature and books, with, as Kretschmer describes, " something pleasantly soft, tender, and lovable, something clinging about it, and yet there is always a light elegiac trait of painful strangeness and susceptibility." Friendly, sensitive, submissive in tests ; very modest yet boyish attitude ; attractive personality. Disagreed feelingly with the other boys in their policy to " thrash out " would-be absconders, because it is " too cruel, they even roar with pain ". Is fairly busy, but has no vigorous energy. Slow to see which boy dirtied the table-cloth and received punishment for it. Unassertive, childlike boy. His letters home are very characteristic : intelligent ideas ; does not want mother to inform brother-in-law about his arrest ; only wants to see mother for one minute ; asks smaller brothers to write to him ; very pleased with letters from home ; religious ; affectionate to brother ; " trust in God, the only sweet thought in this lonely life " ; pleasant dreams just before awakening in the morning, sees one from home at his bed-side, and then when he awakes, " such a depressed, bitter feeling " ; interested in little brothers and sisters ; wants to know what people say about him ; asks pathetically for more letters.

Tests proved this boy's intelligence to be exceptionally good.

Kretschmer says that the hyperæsthetic Schizothyme cannot well be studied in peasants—" Kings and poets are good enough for that." That is why, in this boy's case, the attractive, refined side of a delinquent temperament is more manifest than in the other cases. This boy not only succumbs to bribes and threats outside the reformatory ; in the institution the same methods sometimes seduce him. He is used by the other inmates occasionally for homosexual purposes. From the details given, several of the average leptosome's delinquency disposing tendencies are evident. His love of home and mother-fixation makes the native's last bribe a very effective one. The timidity, fear of possible truth in the native's threats, must have been a strong incentive to continue his illicit activities. The notes in the name of a heavy drink buyer were well planned, as we can expect from the intelligent, introverted, calculative leptosome. His conduct in the reformatory is good, as is the case with most of the timid hyperæsthetic leptosomes. He maintains intimate relations with his people by correspondence and feels himself an exile. His brother-in-law should not know of his disgrace—sensitive ego-consciousness.

The weak self-assertion and self-confidence at the root of such susceptibility to the influence and control of others is displayed in various ways in leptosomes, infantile types and also in weakly muscled pyknics. They have much in common with the " Willenlose " of K. Schneider.[1] They are weaklings. In the reformatory their conduct is usually exemplary, but one can hardly rely on their good intentions. The intelligence, with some pronounced exceptions, is rather on the weak side. When the intelligence is very low, this accentuates the weak self-assertion. In such cases more primitive reactions characterize their behaviour. The weakly intelligence together with the placid, affectively lame, autistic (i.e.

---

[1] K. Schneider, *Die Psychopathische Persönlichkeiten*, Leipzig, 1928, p. 73. The asthenic psychopaths of this author are naturally very closely related to our asthenic leptosomes.

defective sociable contact), self-insufficient, scrupulous-anxious Schizothyme temperament and character in many cases prejudice the correct and accurate judgment of such persons in law court procedures. The following case may illustrate this :—

Case 8.—Age 17. Charged with theft of three Merino sheep (total value £3 10s.). Father, previously convicted of stock theft, owns stock to the value of £90 and has an income of £1 per month as tenant farmer. On this he has to keep seven children. The father is of athletic build, and exercises severe discipline on the children. Brother of father (same build) is a real bull-fighter, who once found a man stealing his sheep and tied him to a wagon without clothes for a whole night in mid-winter. The boy is like a long skeleton, upper spine bent forward, a leptosome of the asthenic kind with the exception that his face is long and thin instead of short-egg-shaped. He has a weak physique, pale colour, sores on his legs and body, deep-set eyes without lustre. His energy is weak and slow, but fairly persistent. He remained seated with his legs crossed when I started to take his measurements until I asked him to stand up. In the motion of his long limbs and in speaking, he is very slow. His intelligence is on the borderline of feeblemindedness. His mental motility is so slow (viscous) that, when given a task in the tests, he sits for a long time without a sign of intention to start, as if he does not know what to decide. When tasks prove too difficult he displays something of an " aristocratic " sulkiness. On the sports field quiet and unsociable ; does not partake in sport. The real typical " lame " type—a " slow motion " production. At the swimming pond he starts to dress early so as not to be late for the bell, but does the dressing in the same slow " aristocratic ", unsociable manner, in a secluded corner of the swimming hall. He has no inclination towards girls whatsoever. The letters he wrote also fit into the " lame " picture with " a sensitive core ". He has a weak, large handwriting, hopeless spelling, and incoherent ideas. Writes about sores not yet healed. Longs for home and letters. (Parents never wrote to him.) Father should send a petition to the authorities to reprieve him because he is innocently punished. Pathetic style.

My study of the court procedure reveals the following : Boy worked for a neighbour at a ridiculously low wage. His father ordered him to resign this post, which he did. The neighbour was very angry about it, and ordered the

G

boy not to disgrace the farm with his presence again. Some days after this the boy looked for his father's missing horses on this neighbour's farm, and, as a native boy (12 years) declared in court, drove some of the neighbour's sheep with him. There were no other eye-witnesses, and the neighbour did not ascertain what happened to the sheep, but immediately reported the boy. The sheep driven away were lean old ewes specially tended after in the neighbour's yard, because they were too weak to go with the flock. All the circumstances convinced me that, if the sheep had been stolen at all, the father had something to do with it, because in a previous charge the father was also implicated (stock theft). When I touched the point in the interview, the cold, " aristocratic," lame, dry picture changed. Tears came to his eyes abundantly when he declared he was not guilty. His report tallied with the court details in all respects, except, of course, that he did not drive the sheep away. " S. (the neighbour) will get his day. God's justice will know that he charged me only because I would no longer work for him." The wounded sense of ethico-religious honour is a vivid, bitter feeling complex in the lame emotional life. Even while he was explaining all this, he sat motionless, his legs crossed, the one hanging over the other like a monkey-rope down a tree.

We see in this boy what Kretschmer has described so fittingly. As soon as we come into close personal contact with the Schizoids, who are poor in affective response, " we find very frequently, behind the affectless, numbed exterior, in the innermost sanctuary, a tender personality nucleus with the most vulnerable nervous sensitivity, which has withdrawn into itself." [1]   In the leptosomes of our material, one did not need to penetrate very far to find the vulnerable sanctuary. But quite a few showed the unresponsive, affectively lame exterior, complicated with the timidly retiring attitude to such an extent that the court might have taken it for criminal indifference or a mild form of sulky defiance and obstinacy. This they are not in the ordinary sense of the terms. Kretschmer [2] describes this " Dried and Emotionally

[1] *Physique and Character*, p. 153.
[2] *Physique and Character*, pp. 167, 181, 216. For very brilliant detailed descriptions of these affectively lame variants we must refer the reader to the work of Kretschmer. This affective lameness appears

Lamed type" as "oppressed into silence". "They are astonishingly speechless, almost dumb." "Dry. Constitutionally subaltern." Some of them, he says, are "moss-grown members of the underworld, full of hypochondriacal whimsies". In my material there was one boy who constantly absconded from an industrial school, because, as he complained afterwards, the boys teased him. He was extremely dry, slow and silent. His negative attitude to our friendly appeals and deliberate jokes at first created the impression that he was sulky and semi-defiant for being subjected to our investigation. But afterwards we became more and more convinced that his reserve, negative attitude, silence, etc., were only due to the timidly-nervous crampedness of his feelings. It is a defect in sociable harmony with his environment. Especially in cases with slight athletic admixture, these "affectively lame" individuals may, of course, show occasional obstinacy or nervous distrust, but, as Kretschmer states, "without their anger having anything brutal, or their obstinacy anything stubborn about them."[1]

(d) *The proportion, "sensitivity-dullness" in these leptosomes.*

The statements of Kretschmer quoted above are important both from a theoretical and practical point of view. Particularly the manifestations of the "emotional dullness" aspect of the Schizo-temperament are very important. The manifestation of emotional dullness is of great importance for the real understanding of the Schizo-temperament, and insensitivity or dullness is also very significant for criminology. We note that the polarity "sensitivity-dullness" usually appears in the same individual. All Schizo-personalities have both these

overtly in the expression and general motility. Jaensch describes these manifestations remarkably in connection with his Tetanoid-type: tetany-face, stern, "expression of pensiveness and concern," stiffness, strictly to-the-point, measured precision, and aim-certain movements (W. Jaensch, *Grundzüge* . , pp. 104, 106, 111, 141, etc.).
[1] *Physique and Character*, p. 167.

qualities, some are more inclined towards the sensitivity pole, others more towards the dullness pole. But, according to Kretschmer, the emotional dullness takes different forms. We have endeavoured to show that in the asthenic, and also in the average leptosome of Kretschmer, the emotional dullness manifestations are qualified by the asthenic attitude, or the asthenic form of experiencing, of these people. Accordingly, the emotional dullness takes the following forms : lack of warm emotional reverberation, resonance, with the human environment ; passive, lame indifference ; nervous, timid autism (self-life, introversion, isolation). But this asthenic form of emotional dullness is very different from the passionate insensitivity or insensitive, brutal type. The latter type is active or aggressively insensitive, i.e. a sthenic, expansive, form of emotional dullness. Kretschmer, himself, mentions that these passionate-insensitive Schizoids are usually post-psychotic forms and, moreover, they have " many connections with certain braintraumatic and epileptic syndromes ".[1] Numerous investigations have, as we shall see, indicated that these syndromes have a biological affinity to the athletic and dysplastic constitutions and very little to the asthenic or leptosomic constitution. We shall see too that these relations are also supported by Störring and Skawran's theory that real activity (organic dynamic force) depends on sensations of tension.[2] Their investigations in the light of modern theories on muscle tonus (Lewy),[3] make it probable that these sensations derive from well-toned muscles such as those found in the athletic type and its mixtures. With the presence or absence of large, hard muscles with a good tonus, not only the activity varies, but also the aggressiveness, self-confidence, absence of fear. This is very easily proved : active feelings form an integral ingredient of the sthenic forms of experience.

---

[1] *Physique and Character*, pp. 170, 204.

[2] Störring, *Psychologie*, pp. 223, 241.   Skawran, " Experimentelle Untersuchungen über den Willen," *Archif. f. d. Ges. Psych.*, Bd. 58, pp. 95–162.

[3] F. H. Lewy, *Die Lehre vom Tonus und der Bewegung*, Berlin, 1923.

Moreover, the same neuroglandular functions which are causally related with the development of strong muscles and broad shoulders, etc., viz. adrenal cortex, male interstitial glands, prepituitary, etc., have been found also to be causally related to the masculine psychical qualities mentioned.[1] Leptosomes, who as a type have a different neuroglandular constellation, lack this aggressiveness, self-confidence, passion, etc., to a large extent. Their insensitivity is, therefore, much less dangerous, though perhaps more frequently accompanied by sly and obscure behaviour. Also, their sensitivity does not easily lead to aggressive retaliations, but to further building of attitudes, sensitive sentiments, " Verhaltungen," as they are called by Kretschmer.[2]

In this connection we may mention another leptosome case where the lameness and lack of warm emotional reverberation was very markedly accompanied by the self-insecurity and constitutional subaltern attitude. He could not swim when he came to the reformatory. When the boys discovered his fear of water they decided that drastic exercise in swimming and diving was the only remedy. This extremely lean, long-limbed juvenile of 18 years, however, put up such a pitiful howl every time they tried to make him swim that the aim was relinquished. He was extremely timid, submissive and credulous. If the other boys jokingly ordered him not to eat carrots while working on the lands, he submitted to the arbitrary order and showed extreme fear when found eating a carrot on the sly. He went to ask for tobacco from the officers for the other boys on their command, even though he knew that tobacco was a strictly forbidden commodity. We see that the emotion of fear, or in the milder characterological form of a timid, self-insecure feeling, is, as Kretschmer states, " an almost universal and in pronounced stages a specific characteristic of the Schizoid temperament." [3]

[1] Berman, *op. cit.*, pp. 174, 196, 211, 238, 246. Pende, *op. cit.*, pp. 13, 22, 24, 54, 57.
[2] *Med. Psychologie*, Leipzig, 1930, p. 199.
[3] *Phsyique and Character*, 159.

It seems as if the excitability of the asthenic leptosome (due to the electrical conductivity of his nerves) [1] is shown primarily in the easiness of discharges of nervous energy into the fear-mechanisms. These fear mechanisms may be located in the Thalamus as Cannon [2] believes, or they may be organic and neuro-glandular changes in the body from where the impulses radiate to the cortex (or Thalamus) to be " experienced " as fear.

(c) Cowardly Acts of Delinquency.

In the cases we have quoted so far, it is very apparent that the leptosome, especially towards the asthenic pole, in his method is far from daring, bold, undaunted. Even in many athletics the delinquent acts make the impression of sly, cowardly, calculation, if compared with the love of nerve-racking adventure, undauntedness, and manly frankness of mixtures between athletic and pyknic. We shall see that forethought, carefully worked out schemes

[1] W. Jaensch has verified experimentally that the galvanic excitability of the nerves of the T-type, especially in pronounced cases, is above the average. He has also shown that this is due to a deficiency of Ca-ions and an excess of K-ions in the system. This deficiency of Ca-ions relative to the K-ions corresponds to a hypofunction of the parathyroid glands. The increased excitability of motorical and peripheral nerves is not so high that it could be called a latent tetany, but nevertheless on account of the hyperexcitability of their nerves, Jaensch calls them the T-(= Tetanoid) type. It is important to note, too, that Jaensch found a relatively high excitability and conductivity of motorical and peripheral nerves to be normal in early puberty—an indication of the connection between the early puberty phase and the T-type (*Grundzuge*, p. 78, etc. ; Berman, *op. cit.*, p. 262 ; Pende, *op. cit.*, p. 22).

Störring and his follower, Skawran, have made very intensive introspective studies of " excitement " as a component of feeling states. With regard to types, Skawran (unpublished lectures, Pretoria, 1930) accepts that the leptosome is particularly " excitable ", i.e. subject to a condition of nervousness corresponding to hyperexcitable nerves in an electrical sense.

[2] Cannon, *Bodily Changes in Pain, Hunger, Fear, and Rage*, New York, 1929, p. 346 and 360. The question seems to be mainly : Does the experience of emotions and feelings depend on visceral, glandular, and vasomotoric changes which are innervated (controlled) by the Thalamus and Corpus Striatum ? (the view of James, Lange, Störring, Meumann, etc.). Or, does the experience of emotions depend only on processes (innervative) in the Thalamus, Corpus striatum, without the mediation of visceral vasomotoric and other changes, which do occur parallel with, but are not the causes of, the " experience " of emotions (view of Cannon, Sherrington, etc.)? Vide also Störring, *Psychologie des Menschl. Gefühlsl.*, 1922, p. 53.

and calculativeness are characteristics belonging mainly
to the leptosomes and athletics, though it is also found in
a less systematic form in the " comfortable enjoyer "
variety of the pyknic group. The careful premeditation
of the Schizothymes, as we shall see, is connected with
the tendency to abstract thinking, to well-planned
theoretical systems of the Schizothyme mind generally.
We shall see that in the athletic this premeditation is
done with calm self-confidence. In the leptosome, however, premeditation is also intimately connected with his
natural tendencies to introversion and to his constitutional
fearsomeness, nervous self-insufficiency.[1]

The leptosome will not usually climb through a flat
window before he has ascertained that the flat is occupied
by a woman or an old man, that the owner is not in, or
that there is a means of escape if the worst happens. In
correspondence with the timidity of the asthenically built
leptosome, I have found in intensive studies of evidence
that these types very rarely venture to break into a place
at night-time, unless they are accompanied by others.
The following cases demonstrate this point :—

Case 9.—In a small town four boys broke into eleven
stores and houses to steal edibles, mineral waters, cigarettes,
money, watches, etc., in a boyish, mischievous fashion.
Two were pyknic mix-forms, and two were leptosomes.
Both pyknics were 15 years of age, the one leptosome was
16, the other 17. All the acts were committed in a period
of slightly over a month. Of the twelve counts, one pyknic
took part in all, the other pyknic in nine. The two leptosomes
joined in after the pyknics had started the game. Some of
the burglaries were done in the day-time, others at night.
The leptosomes were not present in any of the night escapades.

[1] Numerous experiments by Enke have supported this view. A
difficult task is approached with extreme care and hesitation, and every
attempt is made to perform it with utmost precision (*op. cit.*, p. 267).
In a so-called suspicion experiment, the leptosomes showed 80 per cent
mistrust, the athletics 61 per cent, and the pyknics 25 per cent. Enke,
especially, emphasizes the tendency to care, reserve, and assurances in
Adler's sense of the Schizothyme (*op. cit.*, p. 267). Athletics and pyknics
have more equanimity and less hesitation (*op. cit.*, p. 268). Identical
qualities have been found in the T-type of the Jaensch school (*Grundzüge*,
p. 126, 141. Cf. also Pfahler, *System der Typenlehren*, Leipzig, 1929,
p. 228).

Of one operation I obtained a good description in the court proceedings : They stole £25 from a school. The two pyknics climbed in through a window (broke the pane and turned the latch), one opened the door and called one of the lepto-somes, who were waiting outside the school yard. The leptosome entered, but immediately came out again, and looked round to see whether all was safe before re-entering. The leptosome soon came out again, and waited outside till the other two came. They gave the leptosome 10s. (out of £25 !).

These burglaries—though severe from a legal point of view—must be looked upon from a puberty-psychological point of view as more of an adventurous, boyish game. But the timidity of the leptosome juvenile compared with that of the mixed pyknic comes out very clearly. A study of the methods employed to obtain what they want, in almost all of the leptosomes investigated by myself, showed cowardly, timid procedures. In a few cases leptosomes broke into the rooms of their relatives (uncles, brothers) when the latter had left the house and property under their supervision. In fact, it is difficult to find in my material instances where forced entrances into places have been made by leptosomes, unless with the help of others or when there was no possibility of being captured in the act. In the large percentage of cases leptosomes are convicted for sneak-thieving or thefts in lonely places :—

Case 10.—Age 17. Stole five fowls from his brother-in-law, and was caught by a coloured man and held till his brother-in-law came. Pleaded guilty and begged magistrate to send him to the reformatory and not to a prison for four reasons, viz. :—

(1) No parents, no home, and no one to look after him.
(2) He was only 17 years of age, and too young for prison.
(3) Committed crime to get money with which to buy food.
(4) At reformatory he would be able to learn some trade.

No institution offences. But previous conviction for theft of bicycle. Could not find work all over Cape Town, so stole bicycle to pedal to Simonstown, where he hoped to get work on a fishing boat. He was arrested half-way, and given twelve cuts with cane on bare buttocks. Likes bioscopes very much (the boy says), and dislikes daily hard work. In physique he is very thin, with very long legs, and in all respects an asthenically built leptosome.

A type of crime very frequently met with in leptosomes is stock-thefts. There are several aspects of stock-thieving (cattle, sheep, donkeys, fowls, etc.) which seem to fit in with the leptosome's personality. It is usually done away from town in the lonely fields. The solitude of the fields seems to appeal to the unsociable lover of nature, which the leptosome is par excellence. Stock-thieving in the field, carefully planned as it usually is by the weakly impulsed, reflective leptosome, does not entail much danger. Especially in South Africa, with its vast areas and untended flocks, which are in many instances not counted daily, such safe opportunities frequently offer themselves. Also, there is no need to accomplish the act in the dead of night, of which the leptosome, as far as my experience goes, is much afraid. It is done in day-time, in the fresh freedom of the open. This is another instance, therefore, of the cowardly crimes of the leptosome.

The more intelligent leptosomes are susceptible to a form of crime which also indicates the sneakish, calculative, unaggressive nature of the crimes of this type. I have very frequently found forgery and uttering in leptosomes. In my material some of the other types were also prone to this, e.g. the " comfortable enjoyer " variety of the pyknic group and some of the athletics, but it was far more frequent in leptosomes.

Case 11.—Age 16. Stole cheque, forged a signature, and tried to pass it. He repeated the same thing three days later. Boy worked as a page-boy in a large sea-port hotel. Was very desirous to go to sea and see the world. (In our spontaneous drawing experiment, he drew Table Mountain and lighthouse, etc., as seen from the waves—vide Fig. 35). For this purpose, he wanted to work in the hotel, where he could perhaps become attached as a valet to some wealthy person travelling abroad. Liked the work at the hotel because it was easy and neat. Did short trips on sea, and also enjoyed trip into the country—preferably alone. Does not like a variety of girls. Was faithful to one girl and would never seduce her to sexual acts. Did not have the heart for that. Is very religious. Often stole small sums of money. Could not resist the temptation; spent the money on clothes and his trips. Never gave his mother any of the stolen money but some of what he earned. Our observations were: Intelligent, neat, artistic, friendly, fairly frivolous, and talkative when with the other boys. His letters show a very sloping hand with long up and down loops. Somewhat depressed in his letters. The school teacher reports that he lacks will-power, is very easily led, very easy-going, timid and shy, and easily hurt; inclined to be depressed; very obedient and neat.

We see clearly that the crime of forgery and uttering is in harmony with the whole temperament. It is the timid, quiet, intelligent, calculating leptosome who is afraid to do things by force. This boy has the love of solitary nature and the quiet of the seas; but he is too timid to travel into the wide world without a wealthy benefactor to safeguard him.

The argument may be brought forward that we dealt with juveniles, but that a similar self-insecure, timid cowardly attitude towards the social environment need not be found in adults. We admit whole-heartedly that it is impossible to transfer our conclusions from a study of juveniles in any of these types to the behaviour of adults. It is quite possible, as we shall see, that age makes the pyknic less emotionally impulsive and more premeditative. In the leptosomes an increase of age will unmistakably increase the self-reliance. Our bio-physiological theory is that the normal athletic constitution is that of the average adult male. From this one should conclude that the male leptosome with oncoming age acquires more of the athletic calm self-confidence with occasional fits of aggressive anger. But from an intertypical, comparative point of view the leptosome will always be far less self-confident and aggressive than the athletic, and the pyknic less systematic and reflective than either of these. The following cases of adult criminals investigated and considered as typical by Lenz and Böhmer, will prove that the cowardly, timid, calculative qualities of the leptosome are just as marked in the adult as we have found them to be in the juvenile.

Case 12.—Eunuchoid-like length of legs, lean built, feministic breadth of hips, as compared with shoulders. Asthenic body-type.[1] At the age of 13, committed to a reformatory for attempted rape of girl of 6½ years of age. When 21 years old he entered a farmhouse where only a deaf woman was present, strapped this woman on to a bed standing in the kitchen, and stole two silver watches and a walking-stick.

Ten days after this deed, he met a solitary woman on a road. He accompanied her for some distance, and then passed her. Twenty minutes later, at a turn in the road, he unexpectedly appeared again, and confronted her with a stick, saying " Your money or . . ." The woman took to flight, crying for help. He pursued her for thirty paces, then suddenly stopped and fled.

This criminal, called " aggressive " by Lenz, commits the cowardly acts of the asthenic. Unfortunately this one and another one of Lenz mentioned by us in para. 21, are not ideal leptosomes. Both of them are heavily flavoured with inter-sexual constitutional factors (length of legs, disproportion between width of shoulders and width of hips, etc.). A third case given by Lenz [2] is complicated by a very weak intelligence. Some of the characteristics of this unintelligent man are certainly more attributable to the asthenic constitution than to the intelligence defect. His " good nature " is the reason why his wife ignores him, his children disobey him, and fellow-workers " push him aside ". Cowardliness, timidity and slyness speak in every picture of the asthenic delinquent.

The following case is given by Böhmer, who believes that the differences between the types are seen more clearly

---

[1] A. Lenz, *Grundriss der Kriminalbiologie*, p. 74. This is the only good general " asthenic criminal " given by Lenz. The others are sex criminals (vide cases, para. 21). But we consider this case to be a decided hysterical, feministic asthenic. The hips, compared with the shoulders, are distinctly feminine. The length of his legs (96·6 cm.) is out of all proportion to his height. The genital hair shows the typical feminine form of distribution. Also psychically hysterical qualities (according to Birnbaum, *op. cit.*, p. 111) very intimately connected with degenerate feminisms are very apparent in Lenz's analysis of the case.

[2] A. Lenz, *op. cit.* Vienna, 1927, p. 149.

in the method in which a criminal performs a crime than in the class of crime committed.[1] For this purpose, he gives a murder-case for each of the three types of Kretschmer.

Case 13.—Murdered a retired gentleman who lived alone, and stole a casket, containing £13, hidden in the old man's bed. The murderer, who was the husband-to-be of the old man's grand-daughter, did it in this way : At 8 o'clock at night he entered the house, hid himself till the light was extinguished, then he searched for the casket in the cupboard and bed of the murdered man. At this juncture the old man woke up, and was seized by the throat with the left hand, and a rag inserted into his mouth. This made him unconscious. With a towel, the old man's hands were shackled, and his legs bound together with a woollen shawl. When the asthenic (leptosome) left the room he first ascertained that the old man was still breathing. The act was obviously performed with the utmost care ; no rough traces of the agent remained. When arrested, he repeatedly denied his guilt. After much pressure, he acknowledged it to his mother, but asserted that he had not intended to kill the old man.

Böhmer, in his comment on this case, emphasizes that the agent acted with great care, that he did not risk his own security, that he thought, calculated (Kombinieren) exceedingly well in the preparation and performance of the act, left no traces behind him, after the act he reassured himself of his own security and in court defended himself well. As is apparent from this typical case, the pre-psychotic leptosome could hardly commit a murder.

Thus far we have accentuated the temperamentally asthenic qualities of the leptosome. Our material seems to have indicated that the psychically asthenic qualities appear in combination with an asthenic physique (in the sense of Kretschmer) and with the leptosome physique generally, in so far as it is free from athletic admixture. In fact, there is but little somatical difference between the asthenic extreme of physique and the leptosome

---

[1] Professor K. Böhmer, " Untersuchungen uber den Körperbau des Verbrechers," *Monat. schr. f. Krim. Psych.*, Heidelberg, 1928, p. 203. Böhmer supports our contentions that an intensive study of the " court procedures " gives extremely valuable typological data.

without athletic admixture. In practice there are flowing transitions, from the extreme asthenic through the normal leptosome, the athletic leptosome, leptosomic athlete to the pure athlete (vide our *Triangle of Temperaments*, para. 58, Figs. 50, 51).

Throughout our exposition we shall notice the previously mentioned increase of sthenic behaviour with an increase of athletic constitutional factors. This difference in the asthenic-sthenic proportions as we move from the leptosomic to the athletic type is of great importance for a correct comprehension of the " sensitive-insensitive " manifestations. Kretschmer calls this the psychæsthetic proportion and makes it the key to the Schizo-mind. But " sensitivity " and " insensitivity " appear very differently in asthenic and sthenic temperaments. " Sensitivity " in the asthenic person manifests as painful timidity, building of further ego-complexes (Verhaltung), introversion, autistic retiring, self-insufficiency feelings, etc. " Sensitivity " in the sthenic cannot appear otherwise than as excitable aggressiveness, epileptoid crises, dispositions liable to retaliation, quick temperedness, etc. Similarly, " insensitivity " in an asthenic framework may appear as lack of emotional response, i.e. dullness, affective lameness, " autistic distance," coolness, inactive coldness, etc., while " insensitivity " in a sthenic framework must appear as aggressive coldness, brutality or also as calm ego-centric self-complacence, cold self-confidence. This is the reason why " insensitivity " in the leptosomic and asthenic physique type is relatively harmless. Insensitivity-sensitivity proportions in the athletic group are much more dangerous. There these proportions manifest as forms of expansiveness. In athletics aggressive tensions [1] provide the psychæsthetic proportions with a dangerous dynamic moment. In leptosomes, however, these proportions only lead further

---

[1] Sensations of tension are, as the school of Störring has found, of strong dynamic moment. These sensations of tension develop from tension and tonus of muscles such as are found in the athletics par excellence. Störring, *Psychologie*, pp. 223, 241, etc. ; Lewy, *Die Lehre vom Tonus und der Bewegung*.

and further into autism and affective crampedness,[1] because they lack the powers of conduction (Ableitungs-fähigkeit), of discharge into skeletal musculature.   In the more asthenic we find the " sensitive developments " (Kretschmer) while in the more sthenic we find the " expansive developments " provided that both asthenic and sthenic experiences are present in each case in different proportion.[2]

The other fundamental 'qualities of leptosomes still to be discussed, such as autism, logical schematicism, sexual peculiarities, etc., are all causally interrelated also with the asthenic form of experiencing.   These are all to a large extent aspects of the same fundamental biological structure.   They influence one another mutually in an inextricably interwoven etiological structure.

19. *The Autism of Leptosomes*

" Autism " was coined by Bleuler to express the most characteristic temperamental quality of the Schizo-group. The autistic attitude is one of the three fundamental solutions of the problem Ego and environment—the other two solutions being the asthenic attitude and the sthenic attitude.   The autistic solution is primarily the privilege of passive and weakly impulsed Schizoids.   Autism is given by Kretschmer as the opposite of extraverted, realism, sociability, and of frankness.   In positive terms it is ego-isolation, self-life, inward-directedness, reserve ; " the construction of an isolated individual zone, an inner reality-foreign, dream-, idea-, or principle-world, an equanimous or sensitive retiring from the mass of fellow-beings, or a cool mixing with them without inner rapport." [3]   Autism is a form of splitting ; that is why Bleuler could say, " the Schizoid splits too much, the epileptoid too little." [4]   The concept of autism has very

---

[1] Ewald, " Konstitution und Charakter," in *Monographien zur Frauenkunde und Konstitutions Forschung*, 1928, p. 51.
[2] Kretschmer, *Med. Psych.*, pp. 197, 199, 200.
[3] Kretschmer, *op. cit.*, pp. 157, 221, etc.
[4] Quoted by Delbrück.

much in common with the concept "integration-resistance" applied to their T-type by the Jaensch school. In fact, W. Jaensch sometimes describes this fundamental quality of the T-type in identical words as Kretschmer does his autism.[1] It is against a Schizothyme's or a T-type's intrinsic nature to make friends easily and directly with a new intruder into his self-world. They maintain an atmosphere of aristocratic or nervous distance until their feelers have assured them of the congeniality of the newcomer. Kretschmer and Jaensch mention that this type feels as if "there is a pane of glass between himself and mankind".[2] Jaensch and Kretschmer also agree exactly that the Schizothyme is either unsociable or eclectically sociable within a small closed circle, or superficially sociable without deep psychic rapport. In the latter instance, the relations are formal, "official." This is particularly found in the coolly active, calculators, hard masters, and the military variants nearer the athletic pole of Schizothymes.[3] In the leptosomes we seem to find more of the eclectively sociable who may have extremely intimate, even sentimental relations with their select few (compare cases 7, 23, etc.). The autism and intimate selective friendships of the leptosome Schizothyme can again be compared with the early puberty autism and sentimentally intimate friendships described by Bühler and Spranger.[4] They seem to compensate in such hyper-intimacies for the defective emotional rapport they have with the rest of their social environ-

---

[1] W. Jaensch, *Grundzüge*, pp. 126, 145, 144. Oeser, *op. cit.*, p. 184. The term integration-resistance was first coined by H. Thomas. Vide also Möckelmann, *op. cit.*, pp. 48 and 51.

[2] *Physique and Character*, p. 152, and *Grundzüge*, p. 144.

[3] *Physique and Character*, p. 216. Möcklemann, *op. cit.*, p. 51. Also our expositions in the sequel supports this statement.

[4] There is the most obvious correspondence thinkable between the autism of leptosomic Schizo's and that of the early puberty genetic phase. Cf. Ch. Bühler, *op. cit.*, pp. 53, 71, 75 : "with the introversion is also found a retiring from the environment which is not entrusted with a knowledge of the new inner life, and from which the change is modestly concealed," "and antisocial individualistic wave," feelings of "deep solitariness and isolation, the inner segregation from the environment". Spranger also speaks of "Attention directed inwardly", "great solitariness" of this period (*op. cit.*, pp. 29, 38, 42).

ment (compare cases 7, 23). The eclectively sociable Schizothymes described by Kretschmer (Hölderline type, mother-fixated, sensitive affectively lame type, serene aristocratic type, pathetic idealist), all belong to the hypersensitive, self-insecure, unassertive group, which we have shown to be primarily leptosomes. In these hyper-sensitive Schizothymes, the unsociable, reserved, retiring attitude towards all, except their select few, is—as Kretschmer indicates—a result of their nervous sensitivity, their timidity and their fear of the harsh contacts with the real human environment. Towards the athletic pole when more masculine self-assertion and revengeful compensatory tendencies come into the personality picture, the unsociable retreating attitude may become an aggressive anti-social attitude, or more commonly a masterful, military ascendancy.

The unsociable, lonesome, temperamental qualities of the leptosomes are naturally shown in the nature and methods of their delinquency. We saw that they are very fond of stock-thieving. One of the reasons for this preference was the loneliness of the fields where the animals graze. It may be argued that all criminals would prefer lonely places for purposes of escape of detection. This we also found to be a reason why the leptosome preferred stock-thieving—he is physically a coward by nature (afraid of the dark, etc.). But it cannot be coincidence that the two flat experts we found were both pyknics and the main burglars in towns were pyknic or athletic mixtures or groups led by athletic mixtures. We shall again touch upon this point in later chapters. In previous pages we also saw that leptosomes are very frequently convicted of forgery and uttering. This is usually done without company. In such forgery crimes of leptosomes, they are able to keep the secret from everyone for months on end. Also, in the direction in which the money thus obtained is spent, or in the need which prompted the acquisition of money there are significant features which indicate the love of unsociable, solitary conditions. In one instance of a leptosome, the money is spent on trips into the country or on the sea (case 11). In another case of an athlete-leptosome mixture the money is spent on a camera, clothes and a rifle to hunt with, all of which indicate the fondness of solitary hobbies. We shall find the same unsociable tendencies described throughout the following pages. In their sexual relations, the leptosomes either manifest perversions such as intercourse with infants (paedophily), with animals (bestiality), and less frequently with others of the same sex (homosexuality), or they are very selective, idealistic and intimate in their relations with girls. In the average leptosome a tendency to promiscuity, or sociable mixing with girls, is very seldom found. We shall see that these unsociable or eccentric sex qualities very frequently lead to court procedures, either directly or indirectly. As we shall see, many delinquent forms of compensation, of re-establishing the status of the ego springs from the autistic division between the " I " and the " external world " (Ego-isolation). If we compare these aspects of the Schizothyme's delinquency with that of the Cyclothyme, to be discussed later on, the autistic (inward-directedness, self-life) tendencies of the Schizothymes are very apparent. In many cases we saw that asthenically inclined leptosomes showed an easy susceptibility to the influence of others. Here the association with self-confident companions who dominate or safeguard them is not a sociable association so much as a subordination to the others. Such associations are based on self-insecurity or rational calculations more than on a natural love of sociable relations with fellow-beings. We must also realize that we are dealing with juveniles, many of them just above the age of 16 and some with infantilistic characteristics. Young people are much more sociable than the average adults. It has been verified in many ways that adults generally are more introverted or autistic than children and juveniles.[1] So we should expect to find less unsociable, independent,

---

[1] Whitman, *J. of Abnormal and Soc. Psych.*, 1929, p. 207 ; Pfahler, *System*, p. 202. In early puberty there is a very pronounced introversion (Spranger, Ch. Bühler).

behaviour in juveniles than in adults. If we refer to investigations on adult criminals as given in Cases 13 and 12, the same solitary procedure is striking in leptosomes. Pyknics are fond of " Bauernfang " done in bands, spend their spoils on cabarets, drinking parties, women, etc. These are indications of the sociable, frank " live and let live " characteristics of pyknics as compared with leptosomes.

As Kretschmer indicates, the autistic shutting away from their fellow men naturally involves in many of those who are not simply dumb, the building up of their own world of thoughts and aims. Especially in the self-insufficient hypersensitive personalities a strong antithesis " I " and the " External World " develops. They become very ego-conscious and in every situation the relations between the " reflected self " [1] and the social environment are analysed. " A constant excited self-analysis and comparison," says Kretschmer. The naive self of the infant, which consists mostly of self-assertive feelings, is by this critical self-analysis exchanged for a " knowledge of the self ",[2] sometimes a " knowledge of a present self, aspiring to an ideal self ". This ego of the leptosomes is a product of reflection, of introversion, and as such only starts to appear in the early puberty phase with which we have often previously compared the leptosome. The pyknic self-consciousness, as we shall see later, is more

[1] Professor Znaniecki, *Laws of Social Phsychology*. He explains that the reflected self is the subject's idea of how his fellow-beings see him, think of him. The subject views himself from the standpoint of his social environment.

[2] Up to the beginnings of puberty the child has a naive self-consciousness consisting mainly of self-feelings. " A healthy child does not know anything about his ego, and does not reflect about the ego " (Ch. Bühler, *op. cit.*, p. 44). Stern also says, " The self-consciousness of the child in its early phases is not a knowledge about the self but a feeling of the self, a willing by the self " (*Psychologie der Frühen Kindheit*, 1926, p. 321). The ego-consciousness is a product of puberty and is causally connected with the characteristic introversion of early puberty. But although ego-consciousness as opposed to the naive emotional self-consciousness of the child is a pubertial acquirement, it is nevertheless based on the emotional organic ego of childhood. Vide also Spranger, *op. cit.*, 32, 38 ; Storch, *Der Entwicklungsgedanke in der Psychopathologie*, Berlin, 1924, p. 31 ; Kretschmer, *Physique and Character*, pp. 162, 185, 213, 215, 260.

of a naive self-feeling, not an ego-consciousness. In the Schizothyme the developed ego-consciousness—especially in acts of compensation—makes him do things with the special conscious purpose of raising the status of the "reflected self" in the eyes of the environment. The leptosome nearly always feels himself inferior to others and this inferiority seeks compensation, as Adler has so much accentuated in his works. In the asthenic group the self-insufficiency seems to be rather passive. But in the physically well-developed leptosome with more self-assertion, the asthenic consciousness, i.e. the self-insufficiency consciousness acts as a "sting"[1] to the sthenic consciousness and we get the "expansive" tendency, the strong compensatory ambition. This mixture between asthenic and sthenic consciousness (form of experience) gives the well built or athletic leptosome a marvellous energy and ambition, unique in its perseverence. These analyses indicate the intimate etiological reciprocal connections existing among the various Schizothyme temperamental qualities : the autism, sensitive timidity, ego-consciousness, tenacity of aim. We shall see further on that the sexual qualities and the Schizothyme's method of thinking are similarly interrelated with the qualities mentioned above. These considerations, based on results of the Jaensch and Kretschmer typological studies, give us hope that these types are not mere systematic classifications but fundamental biotypes.

20. *Calculativeness, Reflectiveness of Leptosomes*

Ewald emphasizes that Kretschmer in his later works has rightly limited the fondness of abstract thinking to the leptosomes and asthenics. In our discussions of some of the typological studies of the Jaensch school, the Groningen school and of Pfahler of Tübingen, we shall again touch on the theoretical implications of the leptosome's fondness of abstract thinking and logical

---

[1] These mechanisms are admirably analysed by Kretschmer, *Med. Psych.*, pp. 196, 199.

systems.   The athletics are also to some extent inclined
to have logical reasons for their behaviour.   Especially,
mixtures of athletics and leptosomes seem to be cool
schemers and persons who rigidly enforce with relentless
severity their rational disciplinary systems.   In these
consequent tenacious rigorists the rational systematization
is applied to active practice.   Their military, dominating,
active spirit cannot bear to speculate idealistically without
any reference to practical action.   Metternich, Frederick
William I of Germany (father of Frederick the Great),
and even Calvin and Schiller were not only abstract
systematizers, they forced their systems into practice.[1]
This practical, active, disciplinary bent corresponds to
athletic admixture in their physiques.   Hoffmann [2]
mentions that Frederick had a robust natural physique
and a remarkable energy.   Besides his logical systematicism
in practical government, he was characterized by epileptoid
passionate fits of anger leading to deeds of violence—all
of which modern researches ascribe to athletic constitutional factors.   Calvin is also an outstanding historical
personality who excelled by long-thought-out theological
systems with an inexorable logic.   But his long athletic
face shows slight athletic admixture, and the rigour with
which he applied his system to social conditions shows that
his ideal-world was not fully severed from his real-world.
Schiller is another logical systematizer ; but his " tenacity,
overwhelming energy and amazing courage " (indications
of the athletic factors are also found in his very long face
and tall, upright body), saved him from a splitting between
his ideal and real practical world.   In Schizothymes
generally, we meet with logical systematism, detailed

[1] Delbrück in a brilliant composition on the character and temperament of Epileptics, where the athletic and dysplastic physique types
predominate, also mentions the classical personality of Frederick
William I.   He says in connection with their practical logical
systematization : " The psyche of the epileptoids is a firmly coherent
unity.   Closely, too closely, connected are impulses, emotions, and
intelligence."   Hegelianism as a practical, systematic, political idealism
is also a brilliant example (Hegel was an athletic).

[2] Hoffmann has made an intensive heredity-biological study of the
temperament and character of these Hohenzollerns (*Aufbau des
Charakters*, p. 130).

planning, systematic calculation. As Pfahler [1] has proved, this characteristic is just as fundamental as the typical emotional and volitional characteristics. But from the above examples of athletic leptosomes in history it appears that athletic constitutional factors dispose to a vigorous application of these systems to concrete practice. These athletic variants combine rational systematization with extreme practical energy, a large amount of disciplinary leadership and self-confident assertion. They are described by Kretschmer under " Cold, Masterful Natures ",[2] the only " average men " group of Schizothymes with active self-confidence and strong practical inclinations. This fact, by the way, is another proof that athletic factors play a relatively small part in Kretschmer's Schizo-personalities.

The logical reflective activity of the more sensitive Hölderlin type or the worldly foreign schemers of the Kantian type are more concerned with idealistic creations wherein these inward-directed temperaments live undisturbed by the harsh contacts with practical reality. These " poor in deeds and rich in thought " types are the objects of Kretschmer's descriptions of the more genial personalities. But also the ordinary medium-minded leptosome found in the reformatory shows a strong inclination to reflectiveness, premeditation, systematic calculation in detail of his future chances. Van der Horst [3] has found that the Schizothymes generally are inclined to plan their futures systematically and care-fully and to live up to their calculations. He found that the Cyclothymes are not inclined this way, " they do not think about the morrow." Pfahler and Enke have shown by experiments that ideas, intentions and images are more perseverative in Schizothymes than in Cyclothymes. This " perseveration " of ideas and intentions (attitudes) leads to a more consequent, reflective, planned behaviour.

[1] Pfahler, *System der Typen-lehre*, Leipzig, 1929. We shall discuss the principle of perseveration in a later chapter.
[2] *Physique and Character*, 1925, p. 215.
[3] Van der Horst, *Ztschrift. f. Neurologie und Psychiatrie*, Bd. 93, p. 356.

In the leptosomes such careful premeditation and planning can therefore be expected for several reasons: Firstly, the systematic, premeditated, reflective procedure is a general quality of the Schizothymes. They are more influenced by intentional attitudes, not so much by momentary attitudes and impulses. It is a natural and easy task for them to reflect on the details of their future schemes.[1] Secondly, the leptosomes being always nervously timid and self-insecure are bound to think before they leap. Thirdly, weakly impulsed as they are, they are not inwardly driven into action by a strong momentary emotional action charge (" acute sthenic crises "). When the aim presents itself to the consciousness of the weakly impulsed persons, there is still ample time to reflect on the sagacity of the scheme. Even though the leptosome is " excitable " or " irritable ", due to the lime insufficiency in his nerves, this excitability does not seem primarily to lead to nervous discharges into the centres concerned with aggressive muscular activity (somatic muscle tensions and tonus). On the contrary the excitations are more prone to discharge into autonomic fear mechanisms giving rise to the characterological timidity and " lameness ", in some instances, excited talking, change of breathing, etc. We have, therefore, strong " intrapsychic activity "[2] in the form of ideational protection measures, with weak " conduction capacity " (overt activity). Also, the

[1] As Störring (*Psychologie*, p. 242) and Skawran (unpublished lectures, Univ. of Pretoria) have shown that attention processes presuppose a volitional act (an " intention ") or an equivalent of an act of volition (an innate attitude). All thinking processes depend on such a preceded " intention ", or a preceded volitional act of attention, which during the actual thinking process remains in the background of consciousness (volitional attitude, " Einstellung," task-awareness, task-intention, determining tendency of Ach). We shall see later on that in the Schizothyme " intentions " or volitional attitudes are more persistent and have a stronger influence on the contents of consciousness than in the cyclothymes. The cyclothyme's thinking is more influenced by feeling-states, by perceptual problems (cognitive integration with the environment) and by momentary attitudes. The Jaensch school, as we shall see, arrives at similar conclusions.

[2] This corresponds more or less to what Ewald calls strong " intrapsychic activity " with weak " conduction-capacity " (Ableitungsfähigkeit)—Ewald, *Temperament und Charakter*, Berlin, 1924. Also Kretschmer, *Med. Psycho.*, p. 199.

sensitivity of the leptosome (due to the susceptibility of his autistically complex ego- and sex-sentiments) does not lead to affective expression or discharges, but, as Kretschmer indicates in the hyperæsthetics, to concealed summations of feelings, and to conscious intensification of the sensitive constructions.[1] On account of their lack of active self-confidence and their tendency to reflectiveness to the last detail, especially intelligent leptosomes may be extremely indecisive, problematical natures.   They see so many shades of possible chances and dangers (especially the latter) in their reflections on the future that they are unable to determine which course to take, and welcome a heteronomic decision for them.   From the foregoing discussions we also see once more the inextricable inter-relatedness of such characteristics as careful reflectiveness, asthenic experiencing and autism (secludedness, self-life, inward-directedness).

Reflectiveness   and   scheming   are   generally   taken to increase with age.   On the other hand, increase of self-confidence with age may counteract the timid calculative-ness of the more youthful.   In our juvenile material we have constantly found the nervous premeditation and careful planning in the leptosomes, colder and calmer (self-confidence) calculativeness in the athletics, but here it was sometimes frustrated by passionate anger or un-scrupulous self-confidence.   In the delinquency of many cyclothymes of our material we have found very little system or premeditation.   Unreflective, impulsive and adequate to the momentary situation are their deeds. Naive, youthful freshness as that of a tropical shower, characterizes the delinquent acts of the majority of our pyknics, most of whom, however, have slight athletic

---

[1] *Op. cit.*, p. 199.   I think it is advisable to keep " excitability " and " sensitivity " apart.   They   are   certainly   interrelated.   But excitability seems to depend primarily on the conductibility of the nerves and the susceptibility of the sympathetic system and fear mechanisms. Sensitivity seems to be mainly due to susceptible ego- and sex-senti-ments (complexes) constructed by the introvert on a basis of self-insufficiency feelings.   With the insufficiency feeling there must be, as Kretschmer indicates, a sthenic " sting " in the form of self-conscious ambition, etc.

or infantilistic admixture. One group of cyclothymes showed some premeditation—the " comfortable enjoyers ". But even here, where one would expect careful searching for " the way of least resistance ", the premeditated schemes were mostly of a rudimentary nature, as we shall see in the respective chapters.

In the cases given on previous pages, it is already obvious how carefully planned the criminal behaviour of the leptosomes is. Stealing from a native hut, because white men would not be easily suspected, is an instance. In such a deed, however, the cowardly timid aspect is more striking. The calculations of the more asthenic leptosomes are all more or less prompted by this constitutional fearsomeness. A better instance of calculation is that of Case 7, where the notes for drink were written in the name of an habitual drinker. In Case 10 the logical scheming is apparent from the tabulated reasons given why he should be sent to a reformatory rather than to a prison. In Cases 22 and 25 to be described, this careful premeditation is very pronounced.

Case 14.—Age 18. Theft of £70 and motor-car. Nearly a month before the act he came with a scheme to two of his friends. (One of them is described in Case 43.) At the end of the month he would cash his employer's cheque for salaries in the usual way, then take the money and hire a car for a day. The three of them could then drive to Port Elizabeth, where he could find work in a garage (he disliked the type of work he was engaged in at the time). Christmas was near, and he suggested that the other two would thus have the opportunity of a joy-trip. Naturally, they were extremely pleased with the scheme. Everything happened as arranged. The schemer even remembered to bring false number-plates for the car, which were duly affixed. (Compare this with the pyknics of the trip described under Case 44, where the number-plates were forgotten.) In the court this boy pleaded for a suspended sentence and offered to repay the amount to his firm if they reinstated him in his work. Unfortunately the other two afterwards confessed spontaneously about another car stolen by them in Port Elizabeth when the first one ran dry. Such silly confessions broke the bond of friendship between these two and the first party. In the reformatory our hero instantly started to plan an escape. The project leaked out, and the three were secretly "thrashed out". First to propose the scheme, he was the last to jump in for his share of the thrashing, because he hoped to the last that the officers might interfere ; and also, his leptosomic timidity may have played a rôle. After this he wrote to his brother that they should get him into a labour colony where he could earn money while in custody. Physically he is a leptosome ; though the length of the face, snub nose, broad shoulders (38 cms.), fair trapezius, and medium muscularity generally shows that he is more on the athletic than on the asthenic side of the leptosome group. The somewhat shallow shining eyes also indicates pyknic influence.

It is interesting to note that although this boy showed great resourcefulness and initiative in his well-thought-out schemes, he lacked the courage to carry them out singly. He always sought the physical and moral support of the other two in spite of the fact that in the long run they generally proved to be shackles. This is a happy confirmation of our contention that the leptosome always lacks real manly active self-confidence. In the case of Professor Böhmer (our Case 13), the excellent forethought, as we have already indicated, is also prompted by timidity and anxiety to safeguard himself.

In view of these considerations it should be expected that leptosomes must be very little inclined towards such a dangerous and in the long run unpaying concern as crime. This would then apparently be in flagrant contradiction with our results because we found 42 leptosomes and leptosomic mixtures in a material of 177 juveniles, i.e. 23·7 per cent. Compare this with the athletics' 25 per cent, the dysplastics' 23·2 per cent, and the pyknics' 22 per cent. They are, therefore, apparently as numerously represented as any other type. I say apparently, because the following considerations will reverse the picture. Many of our leptosomes will probably not risk another conviction, i.e. they are first offenders who have in their unpractical lameness not realized the seriousness of the results. Moreover, leptosomes are probably—for the same reason—more easily captured than the more dexterous types. The main reasons for such a high percentage of leptosomic juvenile offenders are, however, the following :—

(a) It is in this critical period of industrial adaptation that the deficient physical powers of the leptosome tempt him to find another form of income. (b) Leptosomes, more than any other types, are susceptible to disturbing sexual perversions. (c) The susceptibility to influence also counts strongly against leptosomes.

Other authors agree with us that leptosomes are generally less brutal, dangerous, and also less inclined to serious recidivism than athletics.[1]

21.   Sexual Characteristics

(a) General.

This side of the leptosomic constitution is of paramount importance. We have on previous pages repeatedly compared the leptosome with the "negation-period" of early puberty, when the normal adult sexual factors begin to function—the transitional period from infantile to adult sex-life. We have also sporadically touched on physical and mental similarities between elongated eunuchoids and feministic persons on the one hand and typical leptosomes on the other.

In all his works,[2] Kretschmer stresses very strongly the etiological importance of the sexual glands for the disease of the leptosomes, viz. Schizophrenia. Ewald also admits the frequent sexual conflicts and anomalies of leptosomes,[3] and mentions that eunuchs show anxious prudishness and a tendency to live in their own phantasies. (Schizothyme

---

[1] Böhmer, op. cit., p. 206. This is also in agreement with the fact that the leptosomic and asthenic habitus depends on endocrine deficiencies. Peritz shows repeatedly that this type is a combination of the Status-thymico-lymphaticus with the Ca-ions deficiency of a hypo-parathyroid constitution (G. Peritz, Einführung in die Klinik der Inneren Sekretion, Berlin, 1923, p. 244, etc.).

[2] Kretschmer, Physique and Character, 1925, pp. 89, 91, 148, 153, 164, 168, 182, 189, 193 ; Med. Psych., pp. 131, 199 ; Storch, Entwicklungsgedanken, p. 50.

[3] Ewald, Konstitution und Charakter, p. 51.

qualities). Lenz [1] gives some extreme instances of criminal homosexuality and sexual infantilisms connected with leptosomic constitutions. Wexberg [2] indicates that the insufficiency feelings so universal in Schizoid depressions are frequently sexually coloured. Hoffmann,[3] in several of his profound psycho-biological analyses of Schizothymes, found such sexual anomalies at the root of their personality developments. Numerous descriptions by Peritz and Berman indicate that weakly developed masculine sex glands, parathyroid deficiency, and domination of the constitution by the Thymus gland, give the typical leptosomic and asthenic body and temperament.[4] Berman, as we shall more fully discuss in the chapter on the biophysiological bases of these types, indicates the relationship between hypo-sexuality and lime-metabolism which is so narrowly connected with tetany and Schizophrenia. In the brilliant monograph of Kronfeld, one also finds many infantile dysplastic types and a few leptosomes [5] with psycho-sexual infantilisms and homosexuality, etc. From the physical descriptions given by Kronfeld of sexually infantile persons, it appears that none, or very few, could be classed under the athletic or pyknic types of Kretschmer. Many of the single physical characteristics correspond to that of the asthenic leptosome : Weak beard and body hair, slender build, hip-shoulder proportion, weak muscles, increased reflex excitability, etc. Many of the psychical characteristics of Kronfeld's psycho-sexually infantile and homo-sexual cases also show remarkable correspondence to Schizoid characteristics as described by Kretschmer. Kronfeld even states that psycho-sexual infantilism, homo-sexuality and Schizoid have to a great extent common constitutional-biological bases.[6]

[1] Lenz, *Grundriss*, p. 203.
[2] Wexberg, *Ztschrift. f. Neur. v. Psych.*, Bd. 112, p. 549.
[3] *Aufbau des Charakters*, pp. 104, 154.
[4] Berman, *Glands Regulating Personality*, pp. 250, 257, 266 ; Peritz, *Innere Sekretion*, pp. 165, 182, 244, etc.
[5] Kronfeldt, *Psychosexuellen Infantilismus*, Leipzig, 1921.
[6] Kronfeldt, *op. cit.*, pp. 57, 62. Vide also Peritz, *Innere Sekretion*, pp. 70, 245.

In a study of the sexual life (of leptosomes particularly), one should take some of the genetic aspects of the sex impulse into primary consideration. Before puberty the parents—especially the mother—have intimate feeling connections with the child.[1] Puberty makes an end to this and brings the beginnings of adult sexual qualities into the picture. These real sexual impulses appear on two planes, the psychical and physical : as eroticism in a tendency to ideal, sentimental, psychical empathy and identification with members of the opposite sex ; as physical sexuality in a desire for or indulgence in, physical intercourse of some form.[2] The physical and psychical sides of the sexual impulse are usually kept separated by the pubertial juvenile and only gradually fuse to one impulse after puberty. At the outset of puberty the sex-impulse may be very uncertain and indefinite in its aim,[3] sometimes diverging from the natural aim, e.g. the impulse may be towards persons of the same sex or may be towards the own body, or the impulse may, on the physical side, be fully satisfied by masturbation, exhibition, fetishism, etc. In normal personalities, the heterosexual aim of the impulse becomes more and more definite as the individual matures.

(b) Weakness of Sexual Impulse.

What sexual peculiarities (or anomalies) characterize the leptosome temperament ? First, we have found a weak impulse in a number of the leptosomes of our material. Such persons do not experience a strong urge to sexual or erotic relations with others. Case 8 is a typical example. The boy never had any relations with girls and does not feel the necessity of marriage. Kronfeld gives another example of an asthenic leptosome, where the weakness of the impulse and also the infantile elements are clearly shown :—

[1] Kronfeld, op. cit., p. 22. Kretschmer, Med. Psych., pp. 134, 137.

[2] Med. Psych., p. 139. Also Spranger emphasizes very strongly this pubertial cleft between what he terms " eroticism " and " sexuality " (Psych. des Jugendalters).

[3] Kronfeld, Kretschmer, Spranger, etc. Spranger definitely maintains that a type of homosexuality is normal in early puberty.

Case 15.—Age 28 years. Never had sexual intercourse or erections, never masturbated or felt any impulse towards a sexual object. Psychoanalytic treatment without result. Strong hereditary taint. Sexual organs normally built. Puberty started at proper time, but it was without any sexual impulse or sexual activity. Since puberty, nocturnal pollutions occurred every eight weeks, mostly accompanied by a vague dream about children's hands. A child's hand generally made a definite impression without evoking active impulses, however. Somatically a pronounced habitus asthenicus of Stiller. Psychically very dependent, pliable, without initiative, etc.

Such extreme cases are naturally very uncommon and on the somatic side are usually characterized by infantile stigmata. Usually they are not found in the reformatory for sexual delinquency, but, as we have previously shown, because they are easily influenced by a wicked environment and lack the necessary active assertion to adapt themselves to industrial requirements. In leptosomes with a sex-impulse not so extremely weak, it is difficult to determine whether the weak heterosexual manifestations are at all primarily due to the weakness of the impulse. We know that inhibitions and other mechanisms such as auto-eroticism, fetishism, mother-fixation, erotic sublimation, etc., may prevent the natural overt manifestation of the impulse.[1] One of the cases described by us (Case 6), manifests very little sexual inclinations towards girls. But he is extremely attached to his mother and, at the same time, very timid generally. The impulse, in spite of a normal intensity, does not manifest in a normal hetero-sexual way. An extravagant tenderness and submissiveness towards the mother when normal juveniles have launched into full independent life, and the persistence of prudish ignorance about sexual matters, often found in these Schizothymes, indicate their anomalous sex-development. The sex-impulse may be present from very early times, and may have an approximately normal intensity, but it does not develop along normal lines.

---

[1] *Physique and Character*, p. 90.

(c) Pubertial and Infantile Factors in the Leptosome's Sexual Impulse.

We shall certainly be nearer the truth if we state that the leptosome's sexual impulse in some respects retains features of an earlier genetic phase.   Mother-fixation, as we have outlined it above, results when feeling-attitudes, normal in pre-pubertial development, are retained in the post-pubertial sex life.   Many exhibitionisms, fetishisms, paedophily, etc., are, according to Kronfeld, also due to the incorporation of infantilistic components in post-pubertial sex-life.   Auto-eroticism and homosexuality also have affinities with the early puberty phase, when sexual object choice is still indefinite (" playing ") and persons belonging to the same sex form intimate erotic relationships.[1]   It is also obvious that many of these abnormalities in the sexual direction pre-suppose a strong separation between the psychical and the physical aspects of sex-object choice.   Mother-fixation is only possible on a psychical (erotic) basis with rigid exclusion of the physical (sexual) side of the impulse.   Sodomy, masturbation and paedophily, on the other hand, can only be practised on a physical basis with exclusion of the psychical aspect of the impulse.   Now, we know that a strong separation between the psychical (erotic) and physical (sexual) components of the sex-impulse is a characteristic feature of the early-pubertial phase of sexual development. It is interesting to note further that the manifestations of eroticism as described by Spranger, who has made a special study of this component of the sexual impulse, correspond to some of the universal characteristics of Schizothymes.   These are some of his descriptions : Erotic relationships are satisfied with admiration from a distance.   " The desire to physical contact, if it appears, is suppressed relentlessly."   It is a mixture of earthly and religious love as revealed in Dante's " Vita Nuova " to Beatrice.   " Inner shuddering, deep shyness, shame on

---

[1] Spranger, *op. cit.*, pp. 89, 123 ;   Kronfeld, *Psycho-sexuellen Infantilismus*, pp. 2, 22, 26, 62.

account of own insufficiency characterize the eros."
"Autoeroticism is quite normal for this period."
Attraction to members of the same sex on an erotic
(idealistic) basis is just as frequent as heterosexual
attraction.   On the other hand, he believes that during
puberty perversions on the physical plane of sex-life are
frequent, and—during this period—cannot unconditionally
be looked upon as abnormalities.[1] The purely physical
manifestations, especially in these perverse forms, are
experienced by the early pubert and by many leptosomes
with shameful surprise ("amazement and aversion," says
Spranger).   We can very well understand the main
principles of the Schizothyme's sexual development from
these considerations.   The susceptibility of the sexual
impulse on the physical plane to perversions and realiza-
tions in a state of rigid isolation from the psychical supple-
mentations gives rise to a strong sense of shameful moral
insufficiency.   On the other hand, the isolated eroticism
leads to an idealistic sentimental conglobulation of the
"higher elements" of sex, religion and art—so frequently
found in the Schizoid temperament.   Kretschmer describes
the conditions plastically in this manner : "Here stand
I, my ethical personality, and over there the sexual impulse
as something hostile, as a continually disturbing foreign
body."[2]   The development of such traits as prudery,
timid scrupulousness, insufficiency feelings, and also more
active compensations, such as moral rigorousness, religious
fanaticism, may be largely traced to these antinomies in
the form of a disunion between physical sexuality and
eroticism.   It is, therefore, apparent that in the leptosome's·
sex-life infantilistic components are etiologically very
significant.   As far as we can see, all the sexual conflicts
and anomalies of the leptosomes can be reduced to
infantilisms in the sense of Kronfeld : the persistence in
post-pubertial sex-life of partial components found
normally and characteristically in pubertial, early pubertial
and pre-pubertial developmental phases.   Even if these

[1] Spranger, *Psychologie des Jugendalters*, 1926, pp. 110, 121, etc.
[2] *Med. Psych.*, p. 140 ; *Physique and Character*, p. 91.

infantilisms are afterwards overcome with advance in maturation the effects on the temperament of their long persistence seem to be more permanent.

(d) Timidity of Leptosomes in Sexual Life.

We have made special attempts in the interviews and otherwise to ascertain how the reformatory boys behaved sexually towards their environment in pre-reformatory days. The general impression constantly created was that leptosomes are more sensitive, timid and immature at this age than the other types. Only a few of them were entirely weakly impulsed sexually. Many had girls whom they loved and idealized, but very few had had frequent physical intercourse with their sex-objects. Many of the athletics and well-built pyknics, on the other hand, were very well acquainted with sexual matters, contraception methods, and were promiscuously inclined, as we shall see in the respective chapters. The leptosomes, with some exceptions, " have not had the heart " to attempt sexual intercourse, unless after a long and intimate acquaintance. The physical relations may sometimes be very strongly desired, but the inhibitions usually hold the upper hand. Case II described above is a typical example. This is in accordance with the fact that the ideal erotic objects, in these cases mostly girls, are not at the same time the only physical sex-objects. The physical sex-impulse is frequently satisfied additionally by masturbation or in a few cases by perverse practices with smaller children (paedophily), animals (sodomy or bestiality), etc. While the physical side of the sex-impulse detached from the psychic (erotic, idealistic) side finds satisfaction along these perverse lines, the erotic side is expressed one-sidedly in the other extremes. The objects of erotic love are idolized and the sense of self-insufficiency shyness with regard to the erotic objects may be very strong. Erotic relations detached from physical con-comitants of the sex-impulse sometimes lead, as we shall see, to peculiar active submissiveness and other forms of similar compensations.

From these discussions and subsequent analyses of sexual delinquents in the leptosome type, it is evident that there are intimate inter-relations among the various aspects of the leptosomic personality : the asthenic attitude (self-insecure, timid, inaggressive), the autism (shy, unsociable, retiring self-life, introverted) and the sexual qualities of the average leptosome. We may, perhaps, go even further and indicate an intimate relation between these qualities and the leptosome's thin-fibred hair, lean body, receding chin, and thin muscles.

(e) *Leptosomic Sexual Delinquents.*

There were not many sexual delinquents in our leptosome material, and some of these sexually delinquent leptosomes showed obvious dysplastic features. Also, Kronfeld stresses the preponderance of dysplastics in sexual delinquents. The leptosome's sexual abnormalities are rarely so pronounced that his inhibitions are not able to conceal them. Especially in South Africa, where there are fewer possibilities of detection by educational and psychiatrical activities, this seems to be the case. Very few of them actually reach so far as the law court.

We may begin with a few instances of perverse, legally punishable forms of physical sexual satisfaction, and then pass on to some cases where the erotic, mystical, idealistic side of the leptosome's sex-impulse also have led to clashes with social order. Of perverse punishable physical sexual manifestations, the most frequent are relations with minor children.

> *Case* 16.—Age 16. Dysplastic leptosome with some athletic admixture. Repeatedly rubbed the genital organ of his stepsister aged 3½ years with his own organ. Seminal discharge. Then one day in bathroom when his brother of 7 lay down to swim in the bath, this boy got on to him and attempted sexual intercourse with him per anum. Another successful attempt in the same manner was made nine months later. After this the boy made another connection with the little sister, actually penetrating the girl's vagina partially. His mother tried to get him off this perversion but without result.

The foregoing is not an ideal typical case at all. Somatically, the boy is well-built. The muscles of his legs are even strong. His legs are not long compared with his trunk. But he has fairly narrow shoulders and relatively broad hips, a short egg-shape-front face, similar to the leptosome constitution. His more strongly muscled body, as we shall see in later chapters, is probably responsible for his fairly aggressive sexual policy. We have not found a single pure leptosome who made attempts—especially not in sexual matters—by force, or without considerable care. The delicately measured movements which were experimentally demonstrated in leptosomes by Enke are only the manifestation in the motorical field of the constitutional carefulness, timidity, retiring self-insufficiency of the leptosome. In the case (Case No. 17) described below, the constitution is more purely leptosomic and the way in which sexual relations with a minor girl were practised also gives a better example of the leptosome's temperament. A case of paedophily in a leptosome described by Lenz [1] is also in conformity with the opinion just expressed. The man, stimulated to the act by contact with his two daughters of 9 and 11 years respectively who slept in the same bed with him, rubbed his organ against these children. He distinctly declared that neither was force used nor cruelty shown. In fact, as far as we could ascertain from our own material, or from the literature on the subject, pure leptosomes are much more susceptible to masturbation which they nervously conceal from the knowledge of all others than to perverse practices involving partners. [2] In some cases of homosexuality, however, recourse had to be taken to partners. Case No. 16 given above is the only one of our material who was charged for it. Accordingly we are not in a position to judge about this abnormality. Lenz [3]

---

[1] A. Lenz, *op. cit.*, p. 150.

[2] *Med. Psych.*, p. 131.

[3] Lenz, *op. cit.*, p. 112. Böhmer mentions that Weil investigated 300 homosexuals and found 70 per cent to be of a tall lean build which he termed asthenic. *Monatschrift* (1928), p. 201. Vide also *Med. Psych.*, p. 132.

gives a good instance of homosexuality in an asthenic, but this case had extreme feministic somatic characteristics. It should also be mentioned that no force was employed, by that individual who was a typical weakly impulsed, unaggressive loafer, a cowardly calculator and a beggar. It is also significant to note that the extreme homosexuality of the case given by Lenz was only discovered while in prison—so carefully did he conceal it, and so unobtrusively did he practise it in free life. As far as homosexuality is concerned, therefore, our tentative conclusions are the following : if not prompted by strong inter-sexual or feministic constitutional strain, one may expect lepto-somes to be averse to physical sexual practices involving other human-beings even if a strong desire thereto is present. When leptosomes give way to perverse practices involving other persons we usually find the same careful unaggressiveness which characterized them in other delinquent directions. The following case of paedophily of a relatively pure leptosome, admirably illustrates the latter statement :—

Case 17.—Age 19. Charged for incest with a half-sister of 13 years. He asked this half-sister to allow him to insert his penis between her legs for payment. He did not force her, neither did he actually enter the vagina. Medical report states, though, that exterior of girl's organs rubbed by male organ. Seminal ejections took place. He did it three times, paid the girl 3*d.* the first time, 3*d.* the second time, and gave her sweets the third time. It was done in the lavatory. He directly admitted the act when charged. Girl admits that he did not force or hurt her. Boy states definitely that he did not intend real sexual intercourse, and did not penetrate the vagina.

The boy is a typical, mediumly-built leptosome. Good intelligence. Excellent progress in the carpenters' shop. Does something in light sport. In all respects his behaviour is exemplary. Shy and blushes very quickly. Quiet and reserved. Very sensitive. Preferred not to speak to me about this charge. Generous and kind-hearted. Seems to be compensating in various ways for his sexually coloured sense of insufficiency. In his workshop he drew my attention especially to a well-finished-off desk which he had made. He keeps intimate relations with his home by means of letters. The following notes were made on one of his numerous letters : intelligent sequence, intimate and attractive letter to brother ; workshop instructor who is very kind to him will find work for him on his release, he writes ; penitent for paining his late father by his misdeed ; warns brother against bad company, and advocates religion.   Large handwriting, fairly regular.

It is evident that intimate acquaintance preceded the sexual relations, that mutual agreement existed, and that it was no incest, but only a perverse way of satisfaction on a par with masturbation.   We may also, *en passant*, note how compensation tendencies frequently follow in the wake of these perverse sexual practices.

Leptosomes, as mentioned above, will as a result of their autism be more inclined to sexual perversions which they can anxiously conceal from the knowledge of their fellow-beings.   Bestiality (intercourse with animals), a parallel to the already discussed stock-theft, is something of this nature.   Two of our leptosomes (though not pure) attempted this perverse practice :—

Case 18.—Age 16½ years.   Charged for bestiality.   When alone in the field, he unclad himself and in stark naked condition he chased a cow into a narrow river-bed where he tied her horns with a monkey-rope.   From the high ground walls which hemmed in the animal he tried to have carnal connection with the animal.   On several previous occasions he was punished for cruelty to animals, when animals were found driven into narrow places from where they could not escape.   It is extremely likely that he practised sexual perversions on these animals as well.

Physically a dysplastic leptosome, medium height, very lean, and with something of an angular profile.   Very conscientious and careful in his work.   Shy, timid, subordinate, and conduct in the reformatory exemplary.   Has several good conduct badges.   Very quiet and reserved.   Fond of drawing.   In spontaneous drawing he made a very fine " quiet life " sketch with extreme precision.   Is an illegitimate child with hereditary taint.

In this case, even more than in the previous one, it is evident that the dis-union between the psychical (idealistic, erotic) side and the physical sexual side of the impulse —a normal phenomenon in early puberty—persists far into late and post-pubertial development in leptosomes. Physically the impulse is satisfied in perverse forms while the erotic component of the impulse reacts to this by excessive shyness, a strong sense of self-insufficiency and brave attempts at compensation either by idealistic relationships or by excellence in work, art or science. Masturbation is a similar phenomenon to the other physical sex perversions and perhaps most common in leptosomes even beyond the puberty age.[1] As Kretschmer and others indicate, this secret practice frequently is the origin of the fundamental sensitivity of the hyperæsthetic Schizo-thyme and the pathological condition of sensitive paranoia.[2] Because of its secrecy and also because it is not a punishable perversion we could naturally not control masturbation practices adequately. Kretschmer mentions its frequency in Schizothymes Also Hoffmann[3] has analysed a case which is so typical that we must give some of the main features here :—

Case 19.—Age 18. Extreme leptosome. From childhood, fearsome, self-insecure, pedantically scrupulous—a real " mother's boy ", and now still attached to mother. Some-times prayed " Our Father " seventy times in order to influence fate favourably. Ambitious, wanted to be recognized. Thought very hard how he could distinguish himself. All these schemes were frustrated, however, by ideas of possible obstacles. Self-insufficiency and sense of weakness developed. He painstakingly studied forms of mimicry in front of a mirror, by which he could impose upon others. Sexual life developed very early. Erections at the age of 8 years. Sexual phantasies of himself standing naked and other boys touching his body. Shortly after this he took to masturbation, supplemented by these phantasies. Also phantasies of girls touching his nude body. From early times he had a strong admiration for his own naked body. He would pose before a mirror and admire his own form, especially his genital organs. Only lately did female bodies

---

[1] *Physique and Character*, p. 91 ; *Med. Psychologie*, p. 131. Masturba-tion is taken to be a normal process in puberty (Kretschmer, Spranger).

[2] *Med. Psych.*, p. 199.

[3] *Aufbau des Charakters*, p. 153.

begin to attract him, but he has never approached an object of love.   He fell in love easily, but always at a distance. Shyness and bashfulness inhibited all overt manifestations. Ethical scruples and fear make him attempt to suppress the masturbation sometimes, which is then experienced as beastly and horrifying.   He even wished to acquire the art of hypnotizing, to be able to achieve more power over girls.

This case illustrates the following components frequently met with in the leptosome's sexual life : auto-eroticism and perverse physical satisfaction of the impulse by masturbation ; timidity and shyness in the approach of the heterosexual object ; disunion between the erotic and physical sides of the sexual impulse.   The auto-eroticism is very interesting because this is probably connected with the Schizothyme's autism (inward-directed-ness, self-life), and the developed ego-consciousness of the leptosome.   Part of his "reflected self" unmistakably consists of images of the own body.[1]   The auto-eroticism is also very significant because it is very frequent in puberty, as Spranger emphasizes, and therefore is another pubertial vestige in the leptosomic temperament.   This tentative observation should be further investigated and, if possibly confirmed, traced genetically.

It is obvious from this case that the sexual impulse may awake exceedingly early in the leptosomes, but it remains in the pubertial stage of development for a considerable period.   In this form it can hardly be dis-covered directly by the observer because of the secrecy and unnaturalness of the relations both on the physical and erotic idealistic planes of manifestation.   On the physical side masturbation up to and sometimes even beyond the time of marriage, or even only phantasies, may satisfy the impulse.   On the psychical side timid, idealistic and sentimental relationships without the object's know-ledge about it frequently characterize leptosomes.

---

[1] Störring has shown (*Psychologie*, p. 296) that sensations of the own body are important components of the ego-consciousness.   In this case not only organic and pressure sensations, but visual sensations and images, probably bulked largely in the ego-consciousness.

(*f*) *Erotic Delinquences.*

The erotic (idealistic) side of the leptosome's sex-impulse is usually bound up with ethical, religious and artistic ideas, and as such it makes for one-sided idealism in harsh contrast with the perverse physical manifestations. But even the idealism in the leptosome's sex-life sometimes leads to peculiar love-murders. It is a kind of flight into death with the love-object.[1] We know that suicide is very frequent during puberty, especially in the early period of " sentimental yearning ", during the " negation period ". The juveniles are disappointed with themselves and their social environment, lack the practical " affirmative " [2] attitude of late puberty and hanker idealistically and sentimentally for a better world. The average leptosome, as we saw, usually retains some of the effects of this early puberty supersensitivity and super-idealism in his temperament. When, therefore, some of the leptosomes meet with disappointments in sexual matters, they may in extreme cases commit suicide and in passionate idealism seek to retrieve in death what they have lost on earth. In our own material we only have one case and even this one (Case 20) is not a typical one, being probably complicated with epileptoid impulses. But for purposes of theoretical exposition we may not leave this aspect untouched for three reasons : firstly, it indicates the similarity between pubertial suicides and those of the leptosome ; secondly, the typical confusion of erotic and mystical ideas by the leptosome is illustrated ; and, thirdly, it indicates the not very distant connections between the depressive pole of the cyclothyme temperamental range and the hypersensitive asthenic pole of the Schizothyme temperament.

[1] Cf. M. Eyrich, *Blätter für Gefängniskunde*, Bd. 61, 1930. It is interesting to note that McDougall interprets the relatively high percentage of suicides in Nordic countries as a racial innate character-istic. He brings it into relation with the introversion and unsociability of the Nordic. Wm. McDougall, *National Welfare and National Decay*, London, 1921. What is more interesting is that divorce is also in proportion to suicide, so that McDougall even suggests brooding over matrimonial wrongs as a possible explanation (p. 110).

[2] Ch. Bühler, *Das Seelenleben des Jugendlichen.*

Case 20. Age 16. Tall, slender leptosome, with some athletic mixture. Lived with a farmer in Rhodesia, isolated from white people. Late one afternoon he met a native woman in the field. He addressed this woman in the Swahili language, asking her for carnal intercourse. She refused, whereupon he drew a knife with which he stabbed her, saying, " If you don't let me, we shall die together." The native woman escaped, however, and the boy returned in a nervous condition to the farmstead. In the court the boy decisively pleaded " not guilty ", and maintained that he tried to defend the native woman against a native assailant. Previous conviction was theft of money from boys in hostel. The boy has a peculiar tendency to manifest an exemplary conduct for more than a year and then suddenly on a slight provocation to outrage all good expectations. He calls it a " sudden impulse " himself. We are inclined to believe something of an epileptoid basis. In the reformatory he showed a calm, submissive and steady good-nature and much conscientiousness in his work. After about two years he once felt insulted because an officer reprimanded him for drinking some of the milk that he drew from the cows. When the officer came on duty again the boy absconded, broke into the stores, armed himself and committed several serious shop-breakings before arrested.

From the words to the native woman " we shall die together ", we see something of the mystical mixing-up of the sexual impulse in some of the Schizoids. Our material was too young to manifest many cases of religious-sexual conglobulation in the sense that persons attempt to attain their ends in death. Weissenrieder gives a brilliant example of such a case. The main features of the case may be summarized thus :—

Case 21.—Age 24. Typical asthenic leptosomic body type. Medium scholastic abilities ; wanted to be a teacher or sales-man, but funds insufficient. Became factory-worker, tried to take private classes. Very pessimistic, does not see any value in life. Serious attempts at suicide when 19 and 21 years old. Generally peaceful, quiet, introvert, and ponder-some. This shy retiring leptosome, in spite of sexual excitability, first attached himself to a girl when he was 21. Afterwards fell in love with a girl nine years his senior. Discovered three months later that she secretly had sex relations with her employer. Broke off his engagement, but

returned to her. Both of them jealous of one another.
Girl reproached him for dancing with another girl, and
teasingly threatened to marry another person. Her
unfaithfulness and threats drove his pessimism to a maximum.
The idea of suicide came to his consciousness, and directly
after this the decision to take his " love with him unto
death ". He throttled the girl and took poison himself.

The self-insufficiency feelings and sensitive ego-
sentiments of the leptosome in this case are integral factors
in the suicidal and murder tendencies. The idealistic
eroticism instead of acting as a deterrent proves to be
an incentive to the act. Vague ideas of a more complete
conjugal felicity in an ideal world are connected with his
sexual problem. Weissenrieder especially mentions that
the above case is a type of puberty catastrophe—another
instance of constitutional similarity between the leptosome
and the pubert. In prison this individual showed a very
good conduct and social prognosis. He prefers solitary
confinement to mixing with the rough criminals. We
shall see that there is very little difference in this person's
behaviour and that of a depressive cyclothyme to be
discussed later. Hoffman [1] has also analysed a similar
case which, judged from his additional characterizations,
must be predominantly leptosome with perhaps slight
pyknic admixture.

Hoffmann's case shows the connection between the
erotic sentimental aspect of the sexual impulse and the
murder ideas more plainly : the young man remembered
that in one of their intimate moments the girl had declared
that she would prefer not to live when he died. These
are fairly extreme instances of Schizoid psychopaths.
But even if, as we believe, there are good grounds to
suspect more than only a difference of degree between
these prepsychotic psychopaths and Schizophrenia,
there does not seem to be a qualitative difference between
these psychopaths and normal temperaments. For
typologies of normal temperaments these psychopaths
present exquisite material. One of the above cases (Case

[1] *Aufbau des Charakters*, p. 151.

20) may already have been subjected to a real " process " and that is why from a normal point of view he is in some respects an enigma. Most of the other cases are, we believe, pre-psychotic personalities and psychopaths, whose analysis, as Bumke says, dissolves into normal psychology.[1]

In the sex-life of a few of our leptosomes we have observed another interesting quality which sometimes leads to delinquency indirectly, and is of great theoretical importance. Promiscuity, as we mentioned, is not frequently found in the leptosome of this age. Even if physical sexual relations are strongly desired and continually pictured in phantasy there are too many inhibitions to realize these desires in the natural course of unmarried conditions. The only opportunity of satisfying the impulse in a natural manner is therefore marriage or another extended intimacy. The result is that these leptosomes fondly contemplate marriage before their limited physical powers have made this possible economically. Another explanation of the early marriage ideas of some leptosomes may be the following : We saw that leptosomes are characterized by perseveration of ideas and especially of volitional attitudes. Such attitudes or intentions in the background of consciousness give system and consistency to their behaviour, and also make continued thoughtful manipulation of ideas of the future comparatively easy. The autism (seclusion, self-life, inward-direction) of the leptosomes also favours constant and repeated ideational presentation of future possibilities. The result is early permanency of sexual relationships, because the future marriage or permanent relation is worked out in detail in phantasy and quickly creates a permanent attitude. Possibly both these explanations are valid in all such cases, because these qualities work together. Other factors also add to the tendency. The selective idealistic intimacies of the Schizothymes certainly predispose these persons to permanent sexual relationships between two persons only. Promiscuous   relationships   with   members   of   the

[1] Bumke, *Die Grenzen der Geistige Gesundheit*, München, 1929.

"common" is averse to the idealistic, "exclusive," or sentimental intimacies of some Schizothymes. Young Schizothymes of the leptosome variety are generally still strongly influenced by the pubertial tendency to "exclusive" relationships. In one of my leptosome cases this early permanency of the sexual object was shown very clearly.

Case 22.—Age 22. Charged for theft by false pretensions. Bought oxen from natives on farms and gave them a false cheque in payment. Asked natives not to cash cheque in the town nearby but to take it to a neighbouring and more distant town. This enabled him to dispose of the stock before his falsehood became public. Previous convictions : Stock theft. Stole sheep from a rich farmer who did not count his stock. Says farmer would never have discovered the theft if the buyer had not informed him.

Boy is a very typical, tall leptosome. Quiet, reserved, and reflective. Weakly intelligent. Has some quiet ambition still. Works hard to learn blacksmithing in the reformatory. The others boys tell me that he is generous and kind-hearted to them, and averse to filthy sex-talk so much indulged in by reformatory boys of his age.

I am inclined to believe him when he told me that in both instances of conviction he wanted to get married, but was too poor, therefore stole to get a footing. He keeps to one girl at a time, and could not satisfy his physical sex desire before he was married. The girls also seem to sponge on him and leave him as soon as he gets into trouble. His letters also fairly reflect his attitude towards girls, as is evident from the following notes : To Sannie, his former girl, grateful for her letter, pleased to hear that she is now getting married, wishes her God's blessing, but warns her not to be in too great a hurry. Asks who the happy man is and when the wedding-day. On a silver-oak leaf the words "Remember me, Sannie". (A month later) to Sannie, asks forgiveness if he had hurt her feelings in the previous letter. Is very sad that she did not reply. Cannot forget her, has tried, but loves her more than ever. Would like to speak to her about his difficulties when he is released, even if she is married. Pathetic, sentimental letter.

This case is of little value from a sex delinquency point of view, but it illustrates admirably how persistent and selective ("exclusive") the love relations of the leptosomes may be. Even after she leaves him, he remains sentimentally attached to the girl. The pyknic would, under similar circumstances, probably have re-adapted himself. Cyclothymes and also athletics, as we shall see, satisfy their sexual desires more naturally without an inhibitory sense of self-insufficiency or unnecessary sentimental limitations or idealistic scruples. Leptosomic Schizothymes are more inclined to " exclusive " persistent relationships.[1] We know that compensations depend on assertive tendencies in a setting of a sense of self-insufficiency, timidity and weakness.[2] The burning eroticism with its idealistic tendencies and self-insufficiency —as it especially is manifested in leptosomes—does not only lead to permanent intimacies but also to self-sacrifice and compensations. Highly developed, hyperæsthetic leptosomes may be dominated throughout a career of indefatigable intellectual activity by self-insufficient erotic ambitiousness and faithfulness to a single sexual object. As such they may be victimized by the sexual object on which they are erotically fixated. One of our more passionate idealists (leptosome-athletic body type) repeatedly stole gramophone records, and on one occasion a violin, to please and impose upon his idealized girls. Those cases of love disappointments leading to suicide and murder, as discussed previously, can also be construed as compensations in an erotic, idealistic, mystical framework.[3]

22. Sthenic Reactions

(a) General Orientation.

We have, so far, dwelt largely on the asthenic qualities of the leptosomic Schizothyme, because the average

[1] This is another instance of correspondence between the early puberty developmental phase and the leptosome personality.

[2] Hoffmann, *Aufbau des Charakters* ; Kretschmer, *Med. Psychologie* ; Schneider, *Psychopatische Personlichkeiten.*

[3] Not only the flight into death, but also the idea of making other persons responsible for a ruined life can be the cause of such suicides (Wexberg, *Ztschft. f. Neur. und Psych.*, Bd. 112, p. 570).

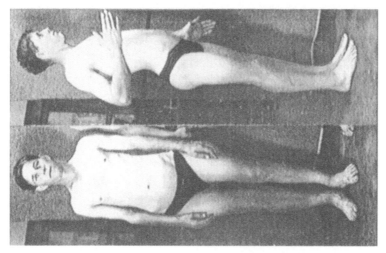

FIG. 31.

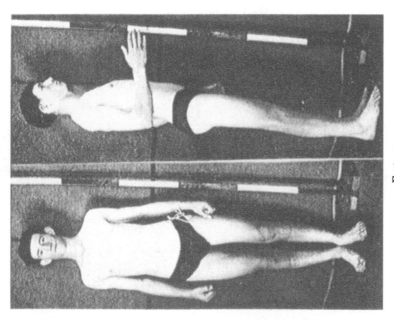

FIG. 32.

[face p. 124

leptosome seems to be more asthenically inclined temperamentally. We saw that the sexual life and the autism of these leptosomes are intimately related with the asthenic form of experiencing. But it also became evident that compensation tendencies are displayed widely in leptosomic behaviour. This is to be expected. Hoffmann, following the doctrines of Adler, indicates clearly that compensations result when a sthenic-asthenic temperamental antinomy exists.[1] It is a consciousness of success, of vindication, of power, in a setting of self-insufficiency. Kretschmer also conceives it in this way : accentuation of certain asthenic partial attitudes as " assurances " against the dominating asthenic experiences. In hysteria we have— as Kretschmer has shown in his classical monograph— a special form of over-compensation.[2] Also, the sensitive developments of the autistic Schizothyme and Schizoid are compensations. Kretschmer shows that in the sensitive development there is a sthenic " sting " of pride and striving in the framework of self-insufficiency feelings. With increase of the sthenic elements (aggressive high-minded self-feelings) we get an asthenic sting in a sthenic setting, and as a result expansive natures. (Jealousy, obsessions, querulants, angry aggressiveness, with fanatical tenacity.) The pure asthenic reaction type is passive, parasitical and depressed. The real sthenic reaction type is imperturbably self-confident, and optimistic, but the proportions of sthenic and asthenic elements in the mixed temperament give the interesting antinomious qualities which are so much emphasized by Hoffmann, both in pathology and in normal characterology.[3] There are hardly any leptosomes who are entirely asthenic in their attitude towards the environment. There are always possibilities of compensation : the building up of an autistic inner world, the realization of sexual and erotic wishes in phantasy, moral and religious rigorousness, scruples and prudery, are all forms of compensation found particularly

[1] *Aufbau des Charakters*, 1926, p. 117.
[2] *Kretschmer, Über Hysterie*, Leipzig, 1927 ; *Med. Psych.*, p. 182.
[3] *Aufbau des Charakters ;* Kretschmer, *Med. Psych.*, p. 197. Schneider, *Psychopatische Persönlichkeiten*, p. 41, 46.

in Schizothymes. In mentally highly-developed Schizo-thymes, magnificent intellectual activities, characterized by marvellous tenacity are not uncommon.[1]

(b) Compensations in their own small circle.

The extreme craving for recognition which we have seen in a previous case (Case No. 19) may in some cases of asthenic or pure leptosomes lead to vain boasting about their own abilities and intentions and to other delinquent compensations. But it is very typical that such verbal self-assertion or other forms of self-assertion are usually exhibited in their own little circle only. They compensate in their own circle for the lack of recognition they receive generally :—

Case 23.—Age 19 years. Stole small articles from a billiard room where he played snooker. Sent to juvenile hostel for two years. Frequent change of employer, though kept to same type of work—bootmaking. Hostel warden states that he is disinclined to work. Deserted from hostel after a year. In court stated that his girl became pregnant as a result of their relationship (boasting with sexual acts to girl) and that he deserted to marry her. He further stated that his wages £2 10s. per week were sufficient to keep them, and that if the court does not show mercy and let him free to marry, the girl's name would be ruined. Sent to reformatory for remaining year. He and his mother are mutually extremely attached.

Told me that he earned £4 10s. when committed. Likes to dance in modern styles. Preferred to dance with his own girl throughout the evening. Had this girl for over two years. Visited her every night, stayed up to 3 o'clock many times. Good conduct in reformatory. Quiet and timid generally, but very fond of talking to me about his musical ability, his home-life, etc., when sympathetically encouraged.

---

[1] It is an acknowledged fact that the purest forms of Schizothymy as it is found in pre-psychotics are characterized by remarkable industrious-ness and conscientious application. Lepel, " Schizophrenie bei ehemaligen Musterschülern," *Zt. f. Neur. u. Psych.* 112, p. 592, has given instances of such model-scholars almost superhuman in their uprightness and conscientious industriousness. It has also been experimentally verified by Enke. *op. cit.*, pp. 250, 252, 263. Vide also *Physique and Character*, pp. 181, 185, etc. ; Mocklemann, *op. cit.*, W. Jaensch, *Grundzüge* ; vide Gunther, *op. cit.*, p. 180.

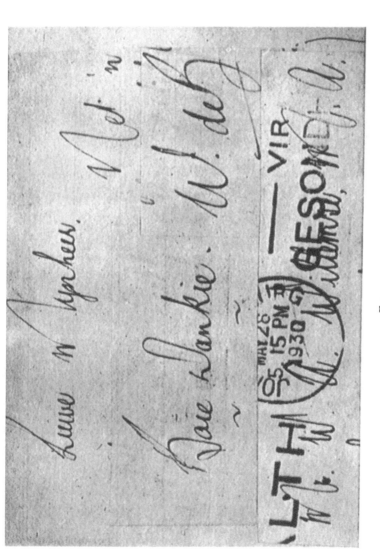

FIG. 33.

[face p. 126

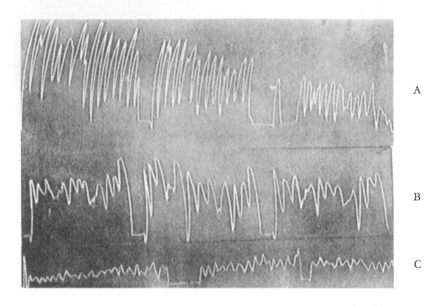

A

B

C

←— direction of writing.

FIG. 34.　A, Pyknic.　　B, Athletic.　　C, Leptosomic.

To some of his corner mates he is also boastful about his past misdeeds and sexual escapades. His letters are very instructive. These are some of the notes on his numerous letters to his " beloved mother " : High flown ideas ; nearly a page on the state of his health " and hopes the same from them ". Ends with " in loving conclusion ". Numerous phrases like the following : " Write soon news from the old city " ; " received and read mother's most welcome letter " ; " regards and thanks to everybody " ; " tons of love to mother." His capitals are very showy and large. On the whole his letters are very ostentatious (vide Fig. 33). Repeatedly writes that " I am going to play on my dearest sister's piano and be at her home with a violin " ; " I have very good taste for all musical instruments " ; " loves letters, violin, brothers, and sister " ; " will accompany his sister's piano-playing with his violin when he returns to the dear home " ; " am not fit for sport, tried once, and hurt my face ".

Very significant from a personality point of view are also the following : He is sly, inquisitive, and cunning in his relations with the boys. Is easily persuaded by others. Strongly disinclined to have himself photographed in a nude form ; but when approached in a friendly manner, he agreed to it, provided that he was taken alone, and not with two others—as was my custom (vide Fig. 31). In the reformatory he made himself an engagement (signet) ring out of brass, with his girl's initial on it. He boasts about the fact that it is the only ring worn in the reformatory. At the swimming pond he is quiet and afraid of cold water ; he never dives, but washes himself on the side of the water, barely wetting his hair. Disdains to mix with the crowd. In practical tests he is very active. Tries to excel. Starts off with a task before he knows the instructions properly, only to be able to finish early.

This is a typical form of compensation by the asthenically built and the pure leptosome. This boy's failure in sport, daily work, normal group-life, are in line with his fundamentally asthenic attitude. But he compensates for this in his sthenic attitude in music, in his showy letters to his mother, his hurry in the practical tests, his exclusive courting of the one girl and boasting with sexual acts to her, his brass engagement ring, etc. All these forms of compensation do not require active self-assertion in the face of a normal environment. There is but little difference between realization of wishes in phantasy and partial realization of them in a small selected circle with a nervous retirement from the open environment.

Some leptosomes, however, compensate for their feelings of self-insufficiency in a less secluded and more openly active assertive manner. They venture to restore the sthenic-asthenic equilibrium by tenacious exertion in the physical field, deeds of bravado in delinquency, disciplinary domination of others, sham boldness in their relations with girls, etc. All of these sthenic reactions can only be understood in an asthenic setting. Skawran has shown that the average well-built leptosomes pull very good ergograms if the fatiguibility of their muscles is taken into consideration.[1] We are inclined to believe with Skawran that their self-insufficiency feelings (termed sensitivity by him) have much to do with the persistent " attitude to overcome the accumulating fatigue ".[2] Other factors not to be lost sight of in this connection are naturally the easiness with which leptosomes generally " adhere to intentions once taken ", and the " perseveration " tendencies already mentioned by Enke, Kretschmer, Pfahler, and by us in previous chapters.[3] The leptosomes of Skawran's triangle-ergogram-type, who correspond to tenacious energy as found in long distance runners, are no pure leptosomes. As previously stated, they are well-built with frequent athletic admixture. It seems to be a general rule—at least in our experience—that sthenic qualities of schizothymes in social, sexual and practical fields go parallel with athletic somatical characteristics.[4] Such features as the following

---

[1] P. Skawran, *Typology of Ergograms.*

[2] A. A. Mumford maintains (*Healthy Growth*, Oxford, 1927, p. 183) that the leptosome type run the danger of overworking themselves (neurasthenia) without knowing it, because in them nervous exhaustion tends to set in without any preliminary signs of fatigue. We consider this interpretation to be incorrect. The leptosome is often inclined to overwork himself, but it is on account of his desire to compensate (self-insufficiency feelings) and his relative weak physical apparatus.

[3] Enke, *Ztschft. f. Ang. Psych.*, Bd., 36, p. 248 ; Kretschmer, *Med. Psych.*, p. 158 ; *Physique and Character*, pp. 130, 175, 259 ; W. Jaensch., *Grundzuge*, p. 454 ; Pfahler, *System der Typenlehren*, pp. 198, 201, 210, 222, 244, 303.

[4] Refer also to our discussion of the connection between leptosomes and depression (para. 39) where we have endeavoured to show that depression depends on asthenic physique and temperamental factors.

are indications of athletic constitutional admixture in the more active, self-assertive and enterprising leptosomes : fairly strong musculature over the whole body or confined to certain parts, e.g. shoulders or legs ; broad heavy shoulders ; massive bones and joints ; extremely great height not due to eunuchoid legs ; height of neck, face, mid-face and head (high head) ; large broad nose ; athletic shape of lower jaw and chin ; large ears ; large coarse hands and feet ; coarse texture of skin ; hard coarse head hair ; secondary hair on face and trunk ; etc., etc. The more pronounced and distributed these somatic character- istics are, the more athletic the somatic constitution becomes. As we shall indicate in other chapters, this conclusion is in line with theoretical considerations. For active self-assertion, very necessary factors are sensations of tension. Skawran and Störring have demonstrated that tensions are important components of the act of will. Now, as we shall later indicate, the consciousness of tension depends upon the tonus and tension of the skeletal muscles. Accordingly, well-developed muscles are presuppositions for active volition.[1] Another theoretical consideration in support of our conclusions is the following : Active self-assertion is a typical masculine form of behaviour ; and, as we shall endeavour to prove later on, the athletic constitution seems to be that of the normal typical male, with the masculine glands (Gonads, prepituitary and adrenal cortex) in a state of hyperfunction.

We have not sufficient material of leptosome-athletic

W. Jaensch, *op. cit.*, pp. 126, 145, 162, 418, 435, has repeatedly emphasized that the pure T-physiological-complex is constantly accompanied by " anxiousness, insecurity, mistrust, depression, unmotivated fear, reserve ". We shall show in the sequel that the pure T-basis almost coincides with leptosomic schizothymy.

[1] According to the finding that epilepsy has an affinity for the athletic physique type, and studies of Mocklemann on the motorical susceptibility of sportsmen, it would appear that well-muscled persons are motorically more excitable than others, i.e. in persons with a good skeletal musculature nervous excitement has a tendency to discharge into the motorical centres rather than into any other centre. Muscular persons therefore do not only have stronger sensations of tension when their muscles receive neural discharges, but their motorical centres are more susceptible to such discharges (vide Bumke, *Lehrbuch*, p. 642 ; Störring, *Psychologie*, p. 195).

mixtures or the space to treat exhaustively all the forms and degrees of sthenic reaction in the schizo-group. The following typical examples must indicate on large lines what we mean.

(c) *Tenacious energy.*

We have naturally not many cases of this socially valuable sub-type in the reformatory who were committed because of their tenacious energy, i.e. the tenacious energy can hardly be a cause of delinquency. But in many delinquent acts of athletic leptosomes the tenacious energy was displayed clearly. One boy of 19 years, accompanied by a smaller boy, rode to a farm at night on a push-bicycle to steal donkeys. He could not find them at the kraal, but followed their spoors into the fields. He found the donkeys and drove them to a farm many miles distant, put them in a kraal, and then fell asleep. This must have involved much energy. Another boy of this type (16 years of age) stole so many things from one place that one marvels how he managed to carry them as far as he did. On another occasion the same boy stole 4 tuning forks, 2 concertinas, 4 locks, 1 footrule, 1 ukelele, set of wire clippers, 1 knife, 1 pair of shoes, 1 bottle of glue, 1 packet of sandpaper, and removed all these articles through the skylight through which he had entered the store. Another boy of this type walked more than 100 miles to a farm of a gentleman whom he knew. When he found this person away he stole 1 pair of leggings, 1 pair of breeches, 1 macintosh, shoes, khaki trousers—all articles required for long-distance walking, of which he was very fond. At the reformatory's swimming pool he manifested indefatigable energy in diving, running and jumping into the water. On top of this he has an amputated heel. He is the best long-distance runner at the reformatory, as well as a good cricketer.

(d) *Self-assertive Mistrust.*

Case 24.—Age 19 years. Stole bicycle ; previous conviction also for theft of bicycle. Six days after committal he absconded by bolting from the farm-party when at work. They all tried to capture him, but he outran his pursuers. He remained at liberty for three months, then stole a suit from his brother and was arrested. In court he stated angrily that he would prefer prison food to that of the reformatory. At the reformatory he is now, however, submissive to his superiors and does good work, although he attempted another escape in broad daylight shortly after the second committal.

Real colour showed to me because he knew that I could not force him. In tests wants to know why we test them. Says defiantly that he is dull, and that everybody knows it. Very suspicious that tests had some evil purpose, and openly stubborn. Tries very hard to excel in the tests, but very difficult to calm his very expansive ego. When measured, very kind appeals and flattering language on my part hardly managed to get him to strip himself. Obstinately and defiantly stated that he could not see any good in our investigations. Said he had to be distrustful because one cannot trust one's own brother. Did not want to have his photograph taken, although 95 per cent of the boys acceded and I tried special courtesy and very humble appeals. The climax came when I started with the interview and asked him in a very friendly tone whether his parents were still alive, and how they were built, etc. He refused defiantly to give me any particulars, stating that nobody had anything to do with his parents. On the sports field he repeatedly stated that he only wished he had my brains and he would be another man. At swimming I once saw that he delighted in pushing a smaller boy under the water.

Somatically: Leptosome with distinct athletic admixture.

The fearsomeness of the average leptosome in these variants is displayed in a much more sthenic form. The boy faces his environment defiantly and not with submissive timidity, but the asthenic setting of his sthenic reactions is very obvious.[1] There is little of the imperturbable, optimistic self-confidence of the pure sthenic reaction type. All his aggressiveness is prompted by the basic sense of insecurity. Though in his attitude

[1] We are now near the real "expansive" reaction group (*Med. Psych.*, p. 196) and there is already some similarity with Delbrück's narrow margined epileptoids and with paranoid querulants (*Stufenstrafvollzug*, 1929, p. 114).

towards my appeals there is much of the " cold despotic type (moral idiot) " described by Kretschmer, my case still falls outside real insanity, i.e. is a characterological variant of the schizo-group.   But Kretschmer's case, with obsessions against his parents and brother-in-law, all of whom he thought guilty of his sister's death, is certainly post-psychotic and as such retained " disease ", or " process " characteristics.[1]

(e) *Rigid Disciplinarian* *(compensations).*

Case 25.—Age 18½ years.   Over a period of a month stole £161 from his employer by changing cheques.   As office boy he wrote out cheques leaving sufficient space in the words-line to insert additional words after the cheques were signed.   Changed 0 into 9, etc.   When charged, he pleaded guilty, and asked for mercy ;   was fatherless, handed his own earnings to his mother ;   wanted money to buy and keep motor-cycle ;   could not bear to allow other boys to give him lifts on their cycles to cricket field—wanted to have his own (compensation).

In reformatory excellent work and ambition in school and on farm.   Keen sportsman.   Tried eagerly to merit praise of officers and very willing to make himself useful in institutional organization and discipline.   Within a year and a half after committal he became the chairman of the Boys'   Representative   Committee.   Proved   excellent disciplinarian and able to control majority of boys.

My observations :   very easily hurt if his authority not recognized ;   nervous sternness towards jokes of boys ; sometimes harsh measures to ensure discipline ; timid and shy of being photographed and measured in nude form ;   ashamed of his brownish skin and lack of beard ;   eager to please head-master   and   very   fond   of   recognition ;   feels   uncertain   in

---

[1] *Physique and Character*, p. 194.   This temperament, described by Kretschmer, developed after puberty as a radical change from the pre-pubertial, conscientious, reserved, serious, and hard-working personality. Puberty was delayed and when it came wrought remarkable changes. This is certainly a case where Schneider and Bumke's criticism that Kretschmer does not differentiate clearly between pre- and post-psychotic characteristics, holds good.   Lepel, *Ztschrift. f. Neur. und Psych.* 112, p. 295, has indicated how often real model scholars and personalities are changed into schizophrenic wrecks in a short time.   It is obvious that such profound changes must for practical and theoretical reasons be looked upon as psychotic and not characterological.   Jaensch also emphasizes (*Grundzüge*, p. 127) that only in pre-psychotic forms are there definite relations between schizoid and his T-type.

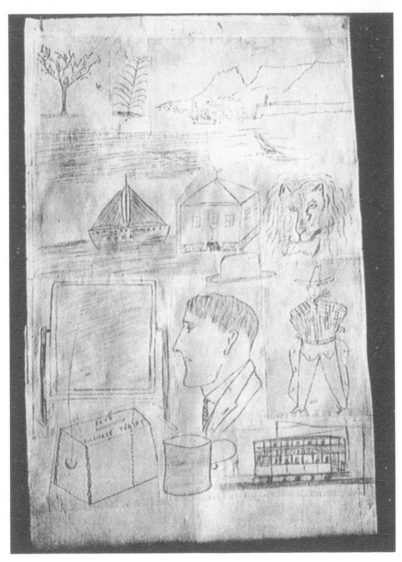

FIG. 35. Spontaneous drawings by Leptosomes, one-third natural size.

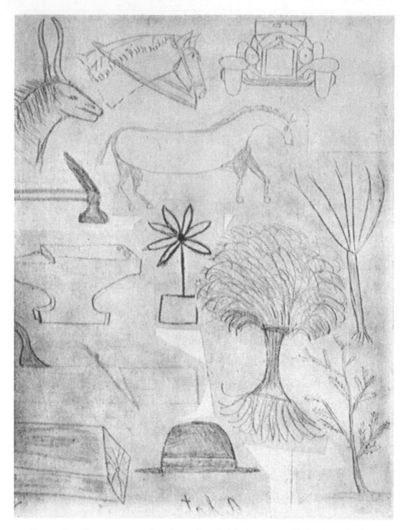

FIG. 36. Spontaneous drawings by Athletics, one-third natural size.

[*face p.* 133

his position ; persistent energy at clipping a long hedge ; unfriendly towards me for a whole week when I reported some of his secret punishments to the authorities ; friendly when humoured. Does not delight in suffering of others, but does punishing for the sake of order and to please officers.

The sthenic reactions are shown in his disciplinary control of nearly 100 boys between 16½ and 23 years of age. In committee meetings he asserts himself drastically. But on careful analysis the feelings of insecurity and lack of self-confidence are very manifest. It is obvious that his delinquent act is a direct outflow of his ambitions, viz. the fundamental struggle to raise his position in the face of subjective insecurity and objective obstacles. It is extremely interesting to compare him with Case No. 27, to be discussed later, who is more self-confident and imperturbable. This latter case is also nearly a complete athlete, i.e. is more sthenic, and not so much stimulated by the asthenic factors calling for compensation. The more completely athletic and sthenic the schizothyme becomes, the less anxious compensation and expansiveness is found and the more calm self-confident assertion.

In connection with organization, discipline and, in general, self-assertion in a leader capacity, it is interesting to note the following observation : The boys have organized themselves into sub-groups, so-called " corners ". These " corners " are for purposes of gardening, conversation, recreation activities and also for many secret practices such as smoking, smuggling, card playing, dirty sex talk, and pictures. Each corner, of which there are about twelve at Tokai reformatory, is led by an influential inmate. Of these corner leaders, I found 6 athletic leptosomes, 10 fairly pure athletics, and 8 well-built or athletically inclined pyknics. There was not one pure leptosome among these leaders. The healthy schizothymes described by Kretschmer under the group " Cold, Masterful Natures and Egoists "[1] will undoubtedly have strong athletic

---

[1] *Med. Psych.*, p. 197.

constitutional features as well.[1] Such descriptions as the following, we feel sure, are not typical for the pure leptosome as described by Kretschmer, but for the leptosome-athletic mixtures and complete athletics: "energetic," "figures of officers and officials," "insensitive to danger, rigid, cold, and born to rule," "exaggerated notion of honour," "they are decisive and take sides," "they feel at home in an atmosphere of commands and stiff beaurocratic discipline," "their passion for rights and discipline borders on narrowness and painful misanthropic coldness," "power-seeking builders of courts, and tyrants of houses," "coldly clever," "unscrupulous and cautious," "sharp formal intellect" (as we find them in lawyers), "ambitious," "successful." These qualities are transitions and mixtures between the excitability-dullness antipoles of the schizothymes on the one side and the boundness (Gebundenheit) -driven (Getriebensein) antipoles of the epileptoids analysed so lucidly by Delbrück,[2] on the other side. The epileptoid characteristics, so common in athletics, are fundamentally of a sthenic pedantic-egocentric nature, as we shall see. This, combined with the schizothyme's autistic idealism, gives the rigorous disciplinarians in moral, social, intellectual and military fields. The schizothyme's excitability in an asthenic setting produces timidity, in an autistic asthenic setting sensitivity and world-flight. The schizothyme's dullness takes the form lame, retired social attitudes of the "Dried and Emotionally-lamed" who are "constitutionally subaltern" according to Kretschmer. Athletic admixture adds to the schizothyme the sthenic egocentric "drivenness" and "boundness", and gradually changes the picture from the asthenic and the sensitive reaction forms

[1] *Physique and Character*, p. 215. This is the only practical, energetic, self-assertive schizothyme (i.e. healthy temperaments) group described by Kretschmer. One could hardly expect to have found it otherwise because "timidity", "weakly impulsed," "constitutionally subaltern," "insecurity in the face of real life" are, according to Kretschmer, some of the universal characteristics of the Schizo-groups. It is probable, according to our discussions, that athletics figured but weakly in the material from which Kretschmer made his classical analyses.

[2] Delbrück, "Gedanken zum Körperbau und Charakter-problem," in *Archiv. f. Psychiatrie*, Berlin, Bd. 82, p. 708.

to the expansive and sthenic reaction forms ; from the subaltern, sensitive affectively lame to the active aggressively cold. The diagram in Fig. 50 will roughly indicate how these transitions and mixtures may be conceived. In normal healthy schizothymes these sthenic characteristics may have great value and attraction. In fact, they characterize the rational, strong, silent man who does not let sentimental factors influence his rationality and principles. But in certain forms of cold brutality found in criminals we reach the psychotic border already. Even if, from a clinical biological point of view, there is only a difference in degree between the socially valuable form and the psychotic forms, it is still very necessary to differentiate clearly between them from a social point of view.

(f) Delinquent Bravado Deeds.

Case 26.—Age 19 years. Stole seven motor-cars, which he took for "joy-rides" and then abandoned. Also stole £30 worth of men's clothing in two counts, smashing very valuable windows for his purpose. All done in the course of ten days. Previous convictions : forgery five years ago and common theft eight months ago. In court he pettifogs about minor details, e.g. tools taken with cars or not. Acknowledges the main charges and asks for mercy.

Observations : Calm, dry humour ; easy-going ; cold and unconcerned letters to his home ; calm and unconcerned attitude to his long sentence and to my investigations ; says his photo will be an excellent illustration for a police paper ; calculative. At swimming pond a real wall-flower, never dived or even wet his hair ; addicted to masturbation and fond of dirty sex jokes ; underhand dealings with fellow-inmates and very boastful about his past misdeeds and his connections with coloured women.

In the interview I discovered the following : Once stood with a few boys on street corner. Discussed criminal acts, each boy boasted about his own. One of them challenged him to steal a motor-cycle standing close by, while the owner went into a building. He reacted bravely, rode round a block, and came to where boys were standing. They patted him on back ; he felt immensely pleased with himself. That was the beginning. When motor-car stolen he enjoys to start off and stop before an admiring crowd, and also likes to pop his head out of the car while he is driving so that people may see him. Likes fine clothes very much. Always wants to carry a revolver with him. Would never shoot with it, but likes people to " know it, though; to know that I am a big man ".

His intelligence is very fair, and he knows much about himself and his aims. At the same time he is fairly pensive. He did not reach further than Standard 5 in school; started on carpentry but often changed work. He is certainly unfit for manual work, and did not have sufficient scope for his intellectual abilities.

Somatically an athletic leptosome (vide Fig. 32). Athletic characteristics : length of face, moulded lower jaw seen in profile, large ears, broad nose, muscular legs, hard head hair. His nearest relatives are very muscular.

This case is of great importance. First, we can clearly see that the heroic reactions are intimately connected with a sense of inferiority. He is very conscious of himself and wants to get recognition of this "reflected self", especially in its physical manifestations. It is not naive self-feelings manifesting in aggressive optimism and unreflective assuming as it is found in the hypomanic cyclothyme. But it is an " ego-consciousness " which, as we have stated previously, is a product of autistic reflectiveness. As Kretschmer says : The antithesis " I " and " The external World ". A constant excited self-analysis and comparison (vide Case 25). He steals motor-cars and clothes to be able to pose consciously before admiring crowds. During his pose he is conscious of himself primarily in the form of images and ideas—not so much in the form of feeling-toned organic sensations. It is important to note his enjoyment of motor-thieving, as compared with that of cyclothymes, to be discussed later. The leptosome enjoys to be seen, to pose as the big man, and would feel very little attracted to "joyrides" if nobody was present to admire him. His " joyrides " are compensations for the lack of the recognition which he desires so fervently (vide also Case 25). The cyclothymes, as we shall see, naively enjoy the " joy-rides " *per se*. The " sensation " of speed, the actual act of controlling the car, i.e. a functional pleasure, as that of a child beating a drum, that is what appeals to the cyclothyme. We have very seldom found schizothymes who steal motor-cars for the sake of " joy-rides " or even for show in the above case. When they stole a motor-car or cycle it was almost always to keep it permanently, or to use it for a definite premeditated aim such as in Case 14. We have found many cyclothymes who steal cars only for " joy-rides ". The above analysis indicates that even where schizothymes, who are so calculative, steal cars for " joy-rides ", their aims are psychologically different from those of cyclothymes. In cyclothymes it is more functional pleasure, playfulness, while in schizothymes it is a compensation, a struggle for recognition by a self-insufficient feeling person.[1] The fundamental difference is that the schizothyme is always so conscious of himself and of his aim. It is, as Kretschmer says, " a constant excited self-analysis and comparison." The cyclothyme, on the other hand, is more naive, child-like, playful. The cyclothyme gives himself up to a project, identifies, integrates himself with his environment or momentary aim in a natural, easy, emotional manner. When he is busy with something his ego and the environment dissolves into one integration-complex, he forgets himself and loses himself. The autistic schizothyme on the other hand is never free from the antithesis " I " here, and over there " the external world ". We have a similar case as that outlined above, where a boy tried to compensate in the following manner : he lifted 3 girls on his motor-cycle, and rode to the police station, where he made a particularly loud noise with his engine to show the girls that he was not afraid of the police. In reality, he is timid towards girls and the rest of his environment. Whether such sthenic reactions take the form of mere phantasy, of unfounded boasting or, finally, of overt heroic escapades depend mainly on the degree of athleticism in the constitution.

---

[1] Vide Enke, *op. cit.*, 251. " I am a little ambitious in such things," " I want to break a record" said the self-insufficient leptosome who looked anxiously and consciously for opportunities to compensate.

SUMMARY OF CONCLUSIONS

1. Within limits the schizo-concept is a valuable working hypothesis.

2. Leptosomes must be differentiated from athletics, the former to constitute the real schizo-type.

3. The asthenic form of experiencing and reaction becomes more and more pronounced as one moves from the athletic leptosome to the asthenic leptosome physique (transitions according to my *Triangle of Temperaments*).

4. Such asthenic mental qualities are manifested in delinquency as : Lack of energy, susceptibility to influences, lameness and timidity, cowardly acts, careful calculativeness, etc.

5. The autism of the schizo-type is manifested in deliquency as a tendency to commit acts solitarily, self-conscious compensations, silent scheming, and sexual maladjustments.

6. The schematicism of the schizo-type is found in delinquency in the form of planned premeditative acts. It is narrowly connected with their volitional attitudes, self-insecurity, etc.

7. The sexual impulse of the leptosome retains many pubertial and pre-pubertial qualities. This is very important from a theoretical as well as a delinquency point of view.

8. Particularly with the increase of athletic factors in their constitutions, leptosomes manifest sthenic qualities in the following forms : compensations, tenacious energy, active mistrust (paranoia), disciplinarianism, and bravado deeds.

CHAPTER V

PSYCHICAL (INCLUDING DELINQUENT) CHARACTERISTICS
OF ATHLETICS

23. *Clinical Studies on Athletics*

The athletics have been grouped by Kretschmer under the schizo-temperament group. Later researches have indicated that not only on clinical grounds are there intimate relations between leptosomes and athletics, but also on experimental psychological grounds. Enke has shown that in the persistence of intentions, endurance of tensions, e.g. in consistent regular pressure on the pen in writing, forethought in the suspicion test, etc., the athletics and leptosomes differ widely from the pyknics.[1] Van der Horst's experiments gave more or less the same results.[2]

But we have already indicated in the previous chapter that there are also wide differences between leptosomes and athletics, especially as far as sthenic-asthenic reaction forms are concerned ; and we indicated that the asthenic characteristics of the leptosomes are intimately related with their sexual, autistic, sensitive and even premeditative characteristics. We may, therefore, also expect significant differences concomitantly with the differences in asthenic-sthenic proportions between leptosomes and athletics in those other characteristics which we have seen to be intimately connected with the asthenic-sthenic proportions. This field is, however, as yet very little worked, and we can only give isolated qualities of delinquent athletics with perhaps a tentative hypothesis of their interrelations.

We may start from what has been found about athletics in clinical researches, because, as we mentioned at the beginning, clinical observations and researches are perhaps

---

[1] Enke, *Zeitschrift. f. Ang. Psych.*, Bd. 36, pp. 237–87 ; *Zeitschrift f. Neur. und Psych.* 108, pp. 645–74 ; and pp. 770–94.
[2] L. van der Horst, *Zeitschrift f. Neur. und Psych.* 93, pp. 341–80.

the best starting-point for more detailed normal psychological studies.[1] Such clinical studies have shown that there is a biological affinity between epilepsy and the athletic and dysplastic somatic constitution. As early as 1914 Wm. Healy[2] wrote this remarkable passage : "No consideration of the epileptic's characteristics is complete without taking account of the peculiar fact that this disease is frequently correlated with premature development and over-development, both of the general physique and of sex attributes. In our study of offenders we have seen some astonishing cases of this. I am not aware that any one has offered an explanation of this unexpected correlation." Healy then gives a few excellent examples of athletic delinquents with epileptic complications. But the problem has been revived in a very systematic manner by the followers of Kretschmer's patho-biological doctrines. Delbrück, after intensive anthropometric studies of epileptics, says : "The epileptic is large, coarse and massively built," "Everything tender, delicate and soft is foreign to the physique of the epileptic."[3] Other investigators such as Grundler, Mauz, Kleist, Forster, v. Rhohden, etc., agree on the high percentage of athletics in epileptic material.[4] The most extensive work is perhaps that of Kreyenberg.[5] He investigated 700 epileptics (500 men and 200 women)

[1] Nearly all modern students of the human mind are of this opinion : Störring, Kretschmer, Ziehen, MacCurdy, Freud, Adler, Jung, McDougall, etc.

[2] W. Healy, *The Individual Delinquent*, Boston, 1914 and 1924, p. 419. It is astonishing to note how little use is made of by criminal psychiatry. In South Africa a case of murder appeared before the Supreme Court. The accused was an outstanding athletic. In spite of this the verdict was given : Accident, subsequent amnesic covering acts performed by the accused as a result of shock of accident. It never occurred to the medical advisers that the deed might have been perpetrated in an epileptoid fit of rage. (This was written 3 months before the same person, van Wyk, killed another man ; for which he was executed. After death sentence he admitted having killed first man (Moller) in a fit of rage ; he had epileptic fits in his youth.)

[3] Delbrück, *Archiv. f. Psych. und Nervenkrankh.* 77, quoted by Kreyenberg. Vide also Delbrück, *Archiv. etc.* 82, p. 708.

[4] Delbrück, *Archiv.* 82, p. 708.

[5] Kreyenberg, "Körperbau, Epilepsie und Charakter," *Zt. f. Neur. und Psych.* 112, pp. 506–48.

according to Kretschmer's somatic typology, and came to the following results :—2·4% pyknics, 12·6% leptosomes, 32·1% athletics, 7·9% lep.-athletics, 45% dysplastics. The "high head"—characteristic of the athletic—was very frequent. The leptosomes amongst the epileptics had a tendency to broadness of shoulders, also a characteristic of athletics, and there were almost no asthenic leptosomes amongst the epileptic material. Kreyenberg has gone further and sub-divided the epileptics into a group with epileptoid characteristics, and a group with epileptic characteristics. He found that the athletic bodybuild has more affinity to the epileptoid characteristics while the dysplastics have more affinity to the epileptic characteristics. Epileptoid he takes, with Kretschmer,[1] as "Rough, defiant, strained ill-humour, explosive anger, violent emotions, alcoholism, reactive absconding"; and epileptic as "Bound, sugary, pedantic, ego-centric, bigoted, dependent, unelastic, circumstantial, sluggish." Delbrück has, however, tried to show that the epileptoid or "agitated", "driven", qualities form a polarity or range of proportions with the epileptic or "boundness", "hypersociality" qualities.[2] In the epileptic individual there is constant shifting between these poles, or, more accurately, the "aggressive agitated", "driven" crises develop on and in the basic epileptic matrix of pedantic, egocentric, dependent hypersociality. The muscularly built epileptics are, therefore, disposed to temporary epileptoid crises in the above sense, though normally they remain in the epileptic characterological state. In this connection it is important to emphasize that just as in the proportions "excitability—emotional dullness" of the schizothymes, "exaltation-depression" of the cyclo-thymes different individuals may differ in their nearness to the one or the other pole, so also may there be differences in the epileptoid-epileptic proportions. Some individuals are more susceptible to the crises than others ; and, as in the case of the other temperamental proportions, some

[1] *Med. Psychologie*, 1930, p. 222.
[2] Delbrück, *Archiv.* 82, p. 708.

individuals may chronically remain near the one or other
end of the range between the poles "agitated, driven
aggressiveness" and "hypersocial boundness".

In connection with the "hypersocial boundness" side
of the epileptoid-epileptic proportion it is necessary to
emphasize that in our athletic material the "dependence,
hypersociality, boundness" did not manifest as submission
to the personal environment. The pronounced self-
feelings, self-justification, sense of superiority, prevents
submission to other persons. It is more a submission to
"fate", to a "godwilled system". In fact, it usually
amounts to self-praise and self-justification by the
indirect route of self-pity and martyrdom pretensions.
Bumke describes the condition fittingly : "All consideration of others is pushed aside. They prefer to speak about
themselves and therewith exhibit a comfortable broad
verbal philosophizing about the self, and a satiated self-
justification. They think themselves more pious,
sympathetic, truthful than all others, have special claims
on heavenly mercy and earthly recognition, etc." "Many
are bigoted and untruthful and all are imbued with the
idea of own righteousness."[1]

It seems as if these tentative characterological formulæ
can be applied to our delinquent athletics. The
proportions "driven-bound" seem to be a valuable
characterological basis for interpreting athletics. The
calm egocentric self-complacent "boundness" usually
forms the matrix on which the driven crises develop. In
many athletics the calm non-emotional matrix of syrupy
talking about the self in an uncritical manner predominates.
In others, isolated aggressive crises disturb the calmness.
Some are continually excited to aggressive reactions and
never remain on the calm matrix for long. But again, in

[1] Bumke, *Lehrbuch der Geisteskrankheiten*, pp. 655, 656. The
traditional religiousness of epileptic characters refers to this. All
clinicians know how unctuously even epileptoid murderers and criminals
always talk of "their" God and "their" Bible. I have found in
private life that another topic of which they are very fond is their
family. The tone is always self-complacent, broad, and adhesive.
"The inherited conviction, firmly rooted in the blood and temperament,
accompanies every judgment and act" says Delbrück.

others there is a functional combination between the two poles.[1] The egocentric boundness to a "godwilled system" is combined with a dominating severity and rigour. This gives us the harsh disciplinarians, severe school-masters, cruel systematic fathers, such as Frederick I of Prussia, and others mentioned by Delbrück in this connection. We shall endeavour to present some of these variants of the epileptoid-epileptic proportions by means of typical cases as we have found them in our researches. In our discussions on the leptosomic temperament, we have previously touched on many of these qualities in a comparative way. We may reiterate that there are many flowing transitions between the leptosomic and athletic temperament to be construed along the lines of our " Triangle of Temperament " (para. 58). With the disciplinarians, to be discussed first, we connect up with leptosomic disciplinarians whom we have already taken to possess some athletic constitutional factors. On the other hand, it is probable that athletic disciplinarians always contain some leptosomic constitutional factors.

24. *Variants of Athletic Delinquents : Masterful Leaders.*

Case 27.—Age 18. Stole revolver from an acquaintance when he saw it in a trunk. Pointed revolver at some of his friends, stating that safety catch was on. Then wanted to try revolver at the river ; placed the revolver in his pocket, but took it out in the street before he reached river. At river one of the boys bent over the bridge to look down into river. Accused aimed at and shot him in the soft part of the buttock. The wounded boy was told not to say anything to the police. Previous convictions : Storebreaking and theft when 14 years of age, theft again when 15. Sent to industrial school till eighteenth year.

In reformatory : Leading sportsman and boxer ; good worker and pupil. Determined, self-confident, relentless leader and supervisor in institutional matters.

My observations : prosecutes trespassers of boys' laws pedantically and relentlessly ; sustained and vigorous energy at swimming, even on coldest winter mornings ; very fond of responsibility ; easily humoured if physical and

---

[1] Delbrück, *Archiv. f. Psych.*, etc., 82, p. 716.

disciplinary abilities praised; bears disciplinary responsibility with self-confident ease; very reasonable when respectfully approached, but at first ill-humoured, defiant, and headstrong in tests; very straightforward even in his letters. In interview he states that he is very fond of firearms and militarism. Very much liked work done at Union's military centre. Fond of exercising and submitting to rigorous discipline. Says he has very little sympathy with weaklings and women. Does not mix with girls, " They are too gentle for me, I am too rough." Somatically, a slender muscular athletic of medium height.

It is very interesting to compare the leader qualities of this boy with the more leptosomic-built boy (Case No. 25), discussed in the previous chapter. The present case lacks the nervous sense of self-insufficiency which characterizes the previous case. In the present case the disciplinary responsibility is sought and borne with self-confident ease. With self-complacency the Ego subjects itself to the impersonal system (" godwilled dependence " of Delbrück) and with self-confident overbearing pedantically subjects others to the same system. Self-assertion, fondness of forceful methods such as firearms, corporal punishment, with very little sympathy for the victims of his aggressive ego, characterize his delinquent acts as well as his institutional activities.[1] Cold rigorism is his key-note. Softness is femininity to him. Delbrück fittingly refers to the rigorous militarism, pedantic activity and narrow views of Frederick William I, the creator of Prussianism, in explaining the " hypersocial "-" aggressive " proportions of the epileptoid characterological forms.[2] It is in this connection that Delbrück says:

---

[1] This fondness of force, guns, and general roughness, was also found by other investigators—Lenz, Bohmer, and Enke—as a characteristic of athletics. Vide also Healy, *op. cit.*, 420 ff.

[2] Delbrück (*Archiv*. 82, p. 716) also gives the following examples: The mathematics teacher who " is severe, pedantic, in general quiet, however, and good-willing. He does not overlook the smallest mistake, not the slightest misconduct ". " Often he appeared with a red head and sullen face. Every one knows that now a catastrophe comes and bad luck to the victim who does not know his tables. The teacher is then ferociously cruel, swears, and punishes." Another case of Delbrück: Orthodox minister, narrow views, "preaches somewhat unctuously, with great emphasis, and a deep serious conviction. In his large family he governs with unlimited force, more feared than loved by the children

" The psyche of the epileptoids is a firmly coherent unity. Narrowly, too narrowly, connected are impulse-life, emotions, and intelligence." There is no separation between their systems and the execution of the systems. The autistic leptosomes have a separate inner-world, to a large extent due to their execution-insufficiency in practical reality. The sthenic ego-centric athletics, however, apply their rational systems *in toto*. So narrowly connected are the volitional motorical consequents to the rational antecedents in the mind of these athletics that they hardly have a separate purely idealistic inner-world; as Delbrück and Bleuler say, "the epileptoid splits too little, the schizoid too much." [1]

We can see from this case and the above considerations that there are flowing transitions from the leptosomic to the athletic personality, from schizothymic to epileptoid. The same flowing transitions occur between the pyknic and the athletic and between the leptosome and pyknic, as we shall see further on. It is, therefore, advisable not to think in terms of pigeonholes but rather in terms of our " Triangle of Temperaments " given in paragraph 58, Fig. 50. We shall see in succeeding chapters that neuroglandular correlates can also be found to fit in with this scheme. Such flowing transitions between " types " must be expected *ex definitio*.[2] But between schizothymes and healthy epileptoids,[3] the connections are much

because he does not tolerate own opinions ; a pedantic piousness," " often enforces his will in unchecked fits of anger." These cases would all have been grouped under the formerly wide denotation of schizoid by Kretschmer.

[1] The too narrow connections between the actions and ideas of the epileptoid may perhaps be explained thus : Möckelmann (*Personlichkeitstypus des Turners und Sportlers*, Marburg, 1929) found experimentally that athletics of the T-type made extensive use of kinæsthetic images in all their mental processes. He also found that such kinæsthetic images were usually supported by kinæsthetic sensations of slight reproduced movements. It is therefore possible that in these people the kinæsthetic centres are more in function than other centres of the cortex ; and it is probable that motor innervations follow more easily from such kinaesthetic centres. These people think in movements, so to speak. Many of these characteristics have also been observed in the Dynaric race, which is largely composed of athletics.

[2] Wm. Stern, *Differentielle Psychologie*, Leipzig, 1921, p. 168.

[3] W. Jaensch, *Grundzüge*, 125, 276, 278.

L

more intimate than between these two types and the cyclothymes. W. Jaensch also corroborates Kretschmer's results in this respect when he makes the epileptoid a sub-group of his T-type,[1] which corresponds psychically, somatically and neuroglandularly to the Schizo-personality of Kretschmer. On the psychological side, E. R. Jaensch's school has found in athletics, sportsmen and gymnasts many characteristics which are typically schizothymic, e.g. " distance " or " formal attitudes " without inner emotional rapport in social contacts; tenacity of intentions; selective friendships; fondness of solitude.[2]

In connection with leaders, it is also necessary to mention that infantiles, weakly-willed persons, self-insufficient leptosomes frequently shelter behind the self-confident athletics, who then play the physical hero.[3] Our cases Nos. 34 and 36 are examples of the latter type. Athletic pyknics, however, are perhaps more inclined to act as leaders than pure athletics, because the latter place less value on companionship.

25. Aggressive Violence

Case 28.—Age 19. Convicted of assault, when drunk, without provocation. Previous convictions : two counts of riotous behaviour, assault, malicious injury to property, contravened motor-car ordinance, known to mix with lowest classes, is heavy drinker. Father divorced from mother because ill-treated her and behaved promiscuously with other women. In reformatory : enjoys a big meal ; very fond of women ; confused consciousness at times ; explosive temper ; lazy at work.

My observations : usually very calm and easy-going ; egocentric, sluggish, friendly, and dependent ; slow but painstaking in tests ; self-confident in attitude to other

---

[1] W. Jaensch, *Grundzüge*, 125, 276, 278.
[2] Möckelmann, *op. cit.*
[3] The strong convictions so firmly rooted in the blood and temperament of epileptoids enable them to impose upon such victims very easily. Vide also Birnbaum (*op. cit.*) for cases of swindling by such self-convinced patent-discoverers. It is remarkable to see how also Supreme Courts can be bluffed with stories of buried treasures and accidents, etc., by such athletic self-convinced murderers.

boys ; explosive temper, smallest provocation makes him blindly angry and then he reacts with violent onslaughts ; is fatalistic towards his own temper, which he is absolutely unable to control. Interview : epileptic fits till the age of 12 ; physician expected that he would become insane ; boy says he is afraid of himself ; drank heavily, and then his temper still worse; assaults people if they only look at him ; does not go in for sport because, if hurt, reacts primitively ; once when tackled in a football match he threw his opponent to the ground and was on the point of crushing his head with a stone ; very frequent sexual intercourse with all sorts, as long as they are females and well-built. Somatically : tall and somewhat stout, heavily built athletic.

This case can be very well interpreted in terms of Delbrück's " driven-bound " proportions. Normally, the boy shows the dependent narrowness, fatalistic sluggishness, but towards his fellows more of a composed self-confidence.[1] It is important to note the latter qualification. In low ebb times his fatalism and " godwilled dependence " has more reference to a condition of things to which all and especially he himself, are subjected, than to his human environment *per se*. This condition of things or " godwilled system " is seen by these people in many forms of manifestation. His own temper and excesses are looked upon as godwilled, " against which he cannot battle." [2] So also a religious, military or disciplinary system may be submitted to as unimpeachable, in a pedantic, narrow, adhesive manner. It is dependence in an adhesive, pedantic and egocentric manner with regard to a super-individual system or condition of things. That is why many authors speak of a " hypersociality ". The pedantic adherence to a religious system or a military

[1] Enke found that in psychotechnical tasks they showed an uncomplicated, semi-fatalistic matter-of-fact attitude, and did not hesitate or say much. They are inclined to do things by brute force. Their most pronounced mental and physical characteristic is massiveness, inertia.

[2] Delbrück, *Archiv.* 82, p. 716. A very good example of such an epileptic delinquent is given by Healy. " I'll kill him, if he is my brother, I'll do it yet. These things come in my mind, Doctor, that's all there is to it, and I go right away and do them. There ain't no stopping to think. When a thing comes in my mind, I just go right ahead and do it, and I don't know why I do " (*op. cit.*, 423).

prussianism is fundamentally related to the fatalistic attitude taken by these people with regard to their own temper; dipsomanic and sexual excesses. In the socially and mentally more advanced disciplinarian, this " hyper-sociality " pole is in a coherent functional unity with the egocentric, aggressive, " driven " pole of the epileptoid temperament.[1] Accordingly the aggressive, driven person enforces the " godwilled system " prussianistically on to his social environment. The dependence and adhesive, pedantic submission of the epileptoid temperament is, therefore, not with regard to the social environment. In fact, a basic characteristic of all athletics in their calm periods, as well as when agitated, seems to be the broad self-complacent discussion of their own virtues, their unparalleled value for the church, home and society at large.[2] Most of them are unable to see the flagrant contra-diction between their broad self-flattering depictions and their intrinsic egocentricity, their prejudiced retaliation on suspected wrongs with the meanest measures and their blind crises with cruel and reckless results. One could not expect it otherwise, because the broad self-flattery, bigotry, and blind driven crises have one thing in common : the utter incapacity to scrutinise the self critically.[3] Every act and judgment is accompanied by strong conviction which is innate and firmly rooted in the blood and tempera-ment (Delbrück).

---

[1] Delbrück, op. cit.

[2] Vide also, Bumke, Lehrbuch, pp. 655 and 656. Healy, op. cit., p. 418.

[3] Delbrück, op. cit., p. 717. In private life I know such an epileptoid woman with a massive athletic physique. She will always turn the conversation to her own egocentric field of interests, and then with syrupy words and broad mimicry accompanied by a deep-rooted convic-tion, elaborate on her industriousness, thrift, mother-love, especially with regard to the step-children whom God called her to keep, religious-ness, regular reading of God's Word, her many sacrifices in all possible good directions. The next moment she will insult one of those very stepchildren with mean expressions and names—and in the same breath tell one of her own children to kiss her father a most happy Christmas. Not long after that she will be able to half-kill both her husband and children, not to mention her extraordinary vocabulary of the most despicable curses thinkable ; and she seems incapable of seeing the flagrant contradictions. One moment tears of compassion, the following hour a violent thrashing scene. In this case there are probably hysterical factors too (cf. Kreyenberg, op. cit., p. 535).

In the case of the boy described above, the aggressive crises are not characterized by the systematic procedure of the cruel disciplinarian. His weakness of intelligence and more primitively impulsive form of reaction may be responsible for this. On the slightest provocation (especially on more primitive levels of stimulation, such as pain-inducement or suspicious-looking at him), he leaves most of his " boundness " characteristics, shifts towards the " driven " pole and reacts with primitive brutality.[1] His aggressions, dipsomanic and sexual intemperance develop as isolated moments in fair contrast with a matrix of fatalistic sluggishness and calm self-complacence. But we have found cases in the literature on the subject and also in our own material where the god-willed dependence and calm self-complacence are persistently over-ruled by the " driven " states of strained ill-humour, aggressive attitudes and active egocentricity. It is possible that more detailed and extensive researches will throw more light on the exact constitutional causes of such persistent " drivenness " crises. It may be that frequency of crises or continued hypertension depend on particular endocrine abnormalities,[2] such as relative size of the pituitary and the sella turcica, or constitutional mixtures such as slight hysterical[3] or paranoid admixture, sexual aberrations, etc. The normally built, pure athletic, according to our

[1] Many authorities (Bumke, Kreyenberg, Healy, etc.) mention that on the slightest provocation epileptics resort to knives or even bricks. It is interesting to note that the same characteristic is found in the Dynaric race, which we have seen to have many somatic similarities with athletics (Gunther, *Rassenkunde*, p. 210, etc.).

[2] Kreyenberg mentions the frequency of endocrine abnormalities in epileptoids. The frequency of dysplastics in epilepsy also point in this direction. Beram has shown that pituitary and sella turcica abnormalities are very intimately connected with migraene and epilepsy, (*Glands*, p. 273, 282), vide also Healy, *op. cit.*, p. 426 ; Bumke, *Lehrbuch*, p. 666.

[3] Hysterical components have been found frequently in athletic epileptics by Kreyenberg. We believe, however, that true hypobulism (Kretschmer, *Über Hysterie*) is foreign to the athletic and leptosomic types. We would agree with Jaensch that hysteria is a sub-group of the B-type. Vide *Grundzüge*, pp. 452, 454 ; and Ewald, *op. cit.*, p. 61. Such athletics, where hysterical factors appear, usually also have feminoid constitutional qualities. This is in agreement with Kretschmer, Birnbaum, etc.

experience is often more disposed to calm, calculative self-confidence than to irritability. They are extremely unemotional and self-contained, so much so that Berman takes them to be the type of self-mastery and calculative intellectuality.[1] It is possible that, apart from their own epileptoid (pituitary, sella turcica) waves, the hyper-tensions of a sensitive-paranoid or semi-idealistic disciplinary nature may be due to leptosomic constitutional admixture, the hypertensions with sexual complications to sexual degeneracy, etc. (vide Case 31). Any neuroglandular irregularity becomes very dangerous in athletics because of their motor susceptibility and the strong dynamic moment accordingly given to such functions.

The most frequent neural or neuroglandular excitement that athletics are subject to is anger, aggressiveness. Though, as we have mentioned, most of them have their calm matrix, crises of " drivenness " develop on this matrix, and the crises are mainly anger or have a strong latent anger in them. The mechanisms of anger are intimately connected with such glands as the adrenals, especially the cortex.[2] These autonomic manifestations and components of the state of anger are certainly controlled by centres in the thalamus and corpus striatum.[3] Whether the consciousness of anger depends on sensations originating from the visceral, vasometer and muscular changes, as Störring, James and Lange, etc., believe, or on the processes in the thalamus and corpus striatum only, as Cannon accepts it, we need not decide.[4] One thing is very probable,

---

[1] Berman, *Glands Regulating Personality*, pp. 192, 211, 246, 247. Vide also Enke's finding about the uncomplicated, semi-fatalistic massiveness, inertia ; lack of emotional attitude ; matter of fact. Kretschmer also mentions that Akromegaly, which depends on a hyper-function of the gland of the athletics (prepituitary), often manifests " a calm, sedate, somewhat torpid and sluggish mental behaviour " (*Med. Psych.*, p. 60).

[2] Berman, *op. cit.*, p. 208. The prepituitary and male interstitial glands are etiologically connected with self-confidence and aggressiveness.

[3] Cannon, *Bodily Changes in Pain, Hunger, Fear, and Rage*, New York, 1929, p. 360 ; F. H. Lewy, *Vom Lehre der Tonus und der Bewegung*, Berlin, 1923, p. 401.

[4] Störring offers a very feasible psycho-physiological modification of the James-Lange theory of emotions in his *Psychologie*, p. 173. Vide also Cannon, *Bodily Changes*, pp. 360, 346.

and that is that sensations of tension (due to muscular tonus and tensions) are an important dynamic constituent of anger. Athletics seem to be extremely immune to the emotion of fear. On account of such absence of fear, and on account of their general insusceptibility to emotions—with the exception of anger—they also seem to have but slight powers of sympathetic empathy (Einfühlung) with others.[1] These characteristics make them very valuable socially as men led by reason and codes of right only.[2] But the immunity to fear, weak capacity to sympathetic empathy and susceptibility to aggressive anger make them extremely dangerous, cold, aggressive criminals.[3] The case described by Professor Böhmer as a typically athletic murderer can, in this respect, be compared with his typically leptosomic murderer (outlined by us as Case No. 13). The essential details of this athletic case are the following [4] :—

> Case 29.—Sailor, released from prison, same evening tried to persuade cab-driver to take him to lonely place. Next evening halted a cyclist on a country road, fired two shots at him, and escaped. The morning after this a farmer tried to catch him. He fatally wounded the farmer in the neck, and fled. A general pursuit followed. He was cornered, and a police officer went to him with raised pistol. Wrestling followed, the athletic freed himself and shot the officer with his own pistol through the heart ; he shot a farmer in the stomach, another one in the leg, and took to flight again. He could not be arrested before he received several wounds, and one of his eyes had been torn out by a bullet.

Böhmer, in his comments on the case, remarks : As in the asthenic, so " also the athletic planfully prepared

[1] Sympathy depends on the capacity to experience an emotion or feeling-state as a result of hetero-induction (McDougall, *Social Psychology*, 1926). A person who is immune to fear, distress, appeal, melancholy, must be incapable of experiencing these feelings in sympathy with others. Another cause of the incapacity to empathize with others is the accepted egocentricity of epileptoids.

[2] Berman, *op. cit.*, pp. 211, 246, 271.

[3] This statement can be supported by many authorities who deal either with athletics themselves, or with pathological syndrome to which this type shows a biological affinity—epileptoid. (Bumke, Healy, Kretschmer, Böhmer, Lenz, etc.).

[4] Böhmer, *Monatschrift*, p. 208.

his act, but his temperament soon gets the upper hand ".
" In the chase he dauntlessly puts his own person at stake."
" There is no sign of fear." " His criminal act is the acme
of brutality and violence, the execution of the act unparalleled in its undauntedness."

A similar case is given by the Austrian authority Lenz [1]
as a typical criminal athletic :—

> *Case* 30.—Short sentences for assault and injury to property
> at age of 17 and 18. In eighteenth year, eighteen months
> hard labour for severe physical injury to several persons
> with a revolver in a robbery fight. Many institutional offences
> for theft. After a short period of freedom another long
> sentence for robbery and violent resistance of arrest. From
> twenty-first year habitual criminal. Many, robberies, assault
> on warder, attempted murder of warder, murder by stabbing
> with a knife, and other acts of extreme violence, are recorded
> against him.

Lenz mentions further in his analysis of the case that
anti-social aggressiveness, excessive drinking, but most
of all, aggressive egocentricity are fundamental qualities
of this case.

Many of us are acquainted with the case of brutal
mass-murder in Düsseldorf, Germany, during the latter
half of 1929, and the first few months of 1930. Judging
from the two available photographs of this man, published
in the *Berlin Tageblatt*, he must belong to the athletic
constitution (vide Fig. 37). The following details taken
by me from newspapers give some idea of this outstanding
criminal :—

> *Case* 31.—Peter Kürten. Age 46. The following gruesome
> assaults are so far known : Killed nine-year-old girl by several
> knife stabs and tried to burn the body; adult man who
> wanted to betray him, fatally wounded with knife stabs over
> temples and neck ; young woman enticed into Rhine
> meadows and skull battered in with a heavy hammer ;
> prostitute woman treated similarly ; five-year-old girl
> literally mazed by knife stabs and also signs of a sexual
> ruse ; two girls of 5 and 14 years brutally stabbed, the head

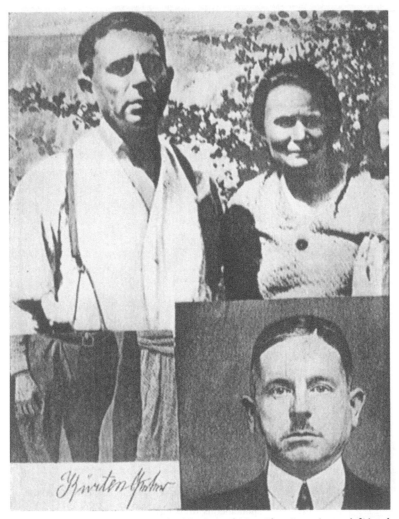

Fig. 37. Note height compared with that of his wife. Inset lower left-hand corner shows hand and lower part of his body.

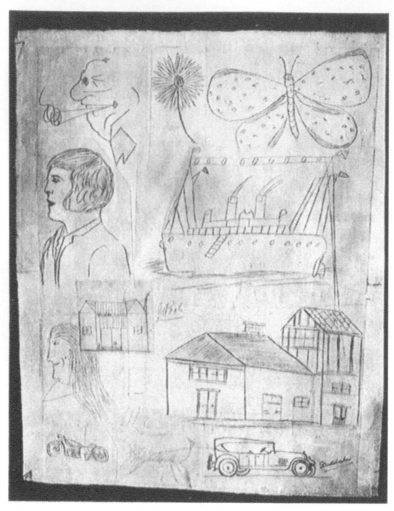

FIG. 38. Spontaneous drawings, Pyknics.

[face p. 153

of the one nearly torn off ; enticed woman into meadows, mortally wounded her with knife stabs ; another woman wounded in same way ; walked with a woman, asked her whether she was afraid in these days of mysterious murders, thereupon she started to run, he overtook her and struck her behind the head with his hammer ; one young woman he met at a bioscope, spoke most lovingly to her, made marriage proposals to her, on a lonesome road attempted indecencies, when the woman refused he got into a frightful rage and was on the point of attacking her violently when passers-by made him desist. Characteristic of his acts were the following : he made sketches and plans, which he attached to trees or sent to the police, indicating the spot of the murder and corpse ; the stabs and blows with his hammer were exceptionally vehement, in one case a knife could only be extracted operatively after 14 days, so force-fully was it driven home [1] ; his wife never knew anything about these murders.

Delinquent from his sixteenth year ; when 19 years old he already terrorized a girl who did not want to accept his proposals, shot at the girl's father with a revolver ; before these murders he had been punished thirty-seven times—on one occasion for forty-six counts of theft—eight times for violence. In prison intelligent, always on the look-out to escape or benefit himself. On one occasion he organized a mutiny among the prisoners, at the same time reported it to the authorities and helped to suppress it. In this way he was pardoned. He very much enjoyed buying the paper in the morning to read about his own gruesome behaviour. After arrest he showed extreme calmness ; he acknowledged his guilt, sometimes corrected the evidences on minor details, and even mentioned a case not known to the police : " I prefer to have my head off directly." Before his arrest he spoke with no sign of excite-ment about the murders to his friend, who did not suspect him, and accurately indicated to this friend the spots where one was committed. In the factory where he worked he was also very unsympathetic and aggressive towards his fellow-workers. His motive for these murders, according to him, was : " I wanted to revenge myself on mankind." By the commission of investigation he is so far taken to be in possession of full sanity.

---

[1] In the South African case of L. P. van Wyk, who killed Tucker, the blows on the skull were so violent that one of the three given would have been fatal. van Wyk is physically and temperamentally a pronounced athletic.

The following characteristics are evident : Aggressive egocentricity ; sexual complications [1] ; very little feelings of sympathy for his helpless victims.[2] But what is also very apparent is the cold, calm, calculativeness, the complete absence of fear or timidity. We shall again revert to this non-emotional calculativeness in athletics. His constant aggressive egocentricity is evident from his driving aim as well : " Revenge on Mankind." The "hyper-social", "dependent", "sugary", side seems to be in complete abeyance. Yet such features as his loving appeals to the girl he wanted to seduce ; his extreme efforts to bury the corpse, to attach indicators to trees, and to notify the police, may have some perverse connections with pedantry and hyper-sociality. His calm, good relations with his wife and his friend, Meurer, are certainly slight manifestations of the " boundness " antipole to the " driven " aggressiveness ; and the fatalistic calmness shown after capture clearly indicates the calm matrix of self-justification on which his aggressive crises developed. The aggressive acts seem to be embedded in astonishing, calculative coldness. Some of these acts even seem to be perpetrated without much anger, as if the non-emotional matrix remained in a coherent functional unity with the aggressive violence and made the deed the more cold and gruesome. As is evident from Bumke's depiction of the epileptoid personality, the pedantic egocentricity, self-justification, lack of consideration for others, constant striving to maintain the " rights " and position of the self with all sorts of means are not only manifested during the aggressive crises, but must also

---

[1] Kürten's father also gave trouble as a result of hypersexuality It is extremely interesting to compare Healy's case (*op. cit.*, p. 427) of an epileptic hypersexual murderer with the case of Kürten. In Healy's case, refusal to conform to his " driven " impulses also gave rise to anger and ghastly murders. It will be interesting to follow Kürten's case with a view to other signs of a psychic epilepsy, which we suspect without doubt. Vide also Bumke, *Lehrbuch*, p. 643.

[2] Compare these characteristics with the general characteristics of murderers, and they are identical (Weissenrieder, *Mitteilungen der Krim. Gesells*, 1928, p. 45). " Gefuhlskalt mit dominanten Verstandesneigungen, Aktivität und Energie, Egoismus, Unempfindlichkeit und Gefühlslosigkeit fur fremdes Leid, Beherrschtheit und Verschlossenheit."

characterize the calm matrix on which the crises develop.[1] These qualities are thus important ingredients of the " boundness " pole as well. On the latter pole these qualities are only displayed in a more calm, self-pitying, or verbal self-glorifying moralizing manner than in the crises of driven, motorical discharges.[2]

26. Undaunted House-breaking and Stealing

Case 32.—Age 14. Convicted of house-breaking and theft with three other boys older than himself. Previous conviction when 12 years old, four counts of store-breaking. In criminal acts distinguished himself by complete absence of fear, took the initiative, although the youngest. Father a heavy drinker. At reformatory undaunted football player, will rush to the ball with bare feet. The following institutional offences are recorded against him : absconded four times ; on one occasion of escape he defiantly broke into store same night to recover tobacco taken from him by officers ; disrespect twice ; gross insolence three times ; theft of food from kitchen ; malicious injury to property twice ; several tattoos ; filthy sexual suggestions twice ; smoking in public. He has now done five years in the reformatory and serves a further sentence for three years. Somatically : Tall, muscular athlete. Would not allow me to test or photograph him.

Case 33.—Age 19. (1) Stole artificial wreath £5 10s. (2) Stole suit-case from station £71 ; (3) Stole watch, riding breeches, leggings ; (4) Stole case of glue £1 10s. ; (5) Stole box of boots £35, from station ; (6) Stole air-gun and bunch of keys. When box of boots stolen, he hired a native with a car, showed him the box, and instructed him to deliver it at his room ; after this he instructed him to fetch a similar box from the station ; the native was detained in the act and the accused arrested.

In reformatory : heavy eater ; bad-tempered, bullying ;

---

[1] Bumke, Lehrbuch, p. 656.
[2] The literary genius of Dostojewsky was also complicated by epilepsy. It is very instructive to note that Dostojewsky submitted to his disease condition with a " godwilled-dependence " ; and yet the egocentricity and broad self-complacence of the epileptoid with regard to his fellow-beings come out as follows : Dostojewsky believed that suffering is the sense of all life, epilepsy is a " morbus sacer ", and he himself is therefore more than others connected with the essence of all being, he is specially called (vide also Kreyenberg, op. cit., p. 530).

fond of boxing and sport ; fond of responsibility ; obscene sex talk. Institutional offences : leaving work without permission, insolence, swearing, disturbing order in school, refusal to do his work, deceitful, etc.

My observations : Quiet, stern in tests ; likes to show his muscles and acrobatic feats ; extreme daring, energy and displayful disposition at swimming pond ; jumps from wall with head downwards into water ; always active manly expression and carriage ; argues well for other boys in boys' court—for secret reward (as I am told). Vicious temper when insulted.

In interview : Wanted to go into navy or army. Very fond of guns, militarism, and discipline. Quarrelled with father and broke off all connections with him; for two years engaged at breaking in horses for a racehorse company ; enjoyed the adventure of stealing, although his first aim was to take things he could use or sell ; quickly left employers when differences agitated him.

Somatically : Athletic, with slight leptosomic admixture.

These cases of athletics speak for themselves. They are in line with the sthenic qualities of athletics already mentioned. Fearlessness and violence against persons and property are the more obvious qualities.[1] In the reformatory or prison the same characteristics dominate their personalities. Especially with slight pyknic mixtures we have found very reckless burglars and even safe-blowers in our juvenile material. It seems as if the pure athletics (without any pyknic admixture) are too coldly calculative to frequently commit themselves to the possibilities of detection involved in reckless house-breaking.

27. Dangerousness and Social Prognosis of Athletic Delinquents

As tensions (and accordingly activity), self-assertion, manliness in males, seem to depend largely on athletic constitutional factors (muscularity, broadness of shoulders, etc.), we are forced to believe that the normal athletic is a valuable social asset. Nevertheless, even within the

---

[1] Enke's results in movement experiments point in the same direction : " They frequently grasped the levers very heavily and did the tracing with excessive force," *op. cit.*, 263. Vide also the cases of Böhmer and Lenz.

limits of normality, pyknic or leptosomic influences always seem to improve the athletic's value for the demands of society. Degenerated athletics or criminal athletics certainly show the worst social prognosis of the three types. Several investigators of large numbers of criminals on the basis of Kretschmer's typology (v. Rohden, Michel, Viernstein, etc.), have arrived at the conclusion that the schizo-group is more disposed towards crime than the cyclo-group and shows the worst social prognosis.[1] They have, however, not differentiated between athletic and leptosomic schizos. Our own studies, as well as those of Böhmer, Lenz, seem to indicate that as far as social prognosis and seriousness of the crimes are concerned, athletics are certainly worse than leptosomes. We have made a systematic study of the improvements of each of the three groups in the reformatories and found that athletic-pyknic mixtures provide the greatest number of clashes with the institutional authorities. The cyclothymes are, as Kretschmer says, "troublesome because of their excessive self-feelings and their tendencies to trump up."[2] But cyclothymes are manageable with tactfulness and humour, and are "not inclined to serious acts of violence, brutality and murder". In the reformatory, the cyclothymes, on account of playfulness, adventure, impulsiveness and excessive self-feelings, are far from submissive, tractable, peaceful and conscientious citizens. The "after-maturation" of cyclothymes with increase of age, however, somewhat improves the above-mentioned faults. Leptosomes, on account of their self-insufficiency are more tractable and submissive, but in many instances unreliable (compare e.g. Case 3). In this connection we may mention an interesting result. In the reformatory at Houtpoort the warden is extremely careful

[1] Böhmer, op. cit., p. 199 : J. Lange, Stufenstrafvollzug Bd. 2, p. 144 ; Viernstein, Stufenstrafvollzug Bd. 3, p. 16 ; Michel, "Der psycho-pathische Gewohnheitsverbrecher," in Mitteilungen der Krim. Biol. Gesellschaft, 1928, p. 85. (In the meantime I have perused all literature in Professor Kretschmer's library in Marburg and ascertained that statistically v. Rohden, Blinkov, and Krasnusckin proved the frequency of athletics in severe crime.)

[2] Kretschmer, Deutsche Jur. Zeit., p. 785.

in assigning corporal punishment, so that the number of cuts given to an inmate during his stay at the reformatory is a fair index of the conduct of such an inmate. On the basis of this we found that athletics are much less susceptible to reformative influences than either leptosomes or pyknics.

The contention that athletics form the most dangerous type of delinquents and are the most refractory to socializing influences is based on a broad basis of evidence. Our own material proves this indubitably. The cases given by Lenz support this contention. Böhmer's [1] investigations on 100 normal criminals from various parts of Germany, gave the following results : 17 leptosomes, 30 athletics, 4 pyknics, the rest mixed. The only three robbers were athletics, similarly the only burglar. Only the athletics were found to be repeatedly convicted before for dangerous crimes. V. Rohden [2] has also found that especially athletics and leptosomic-athletics formed the recidivists and the agents of violence. A fact of paramount importance in this connection is the correlation between the athletic-dysplastic constitution types and the epileptoid syndrome. We know that Lombroso [3] maintained that all crime is a sub-manifestation of epilepsy. We do not accept this broad statement, but future researches will probably show that fits of cold violence, sexual violence, dipsomania, etc., have some connection with epilepsy or, at any rate, with its physiological bases such as pituitary, sella turcica, troubles. Healy gives a few very typical cases of athletic epileptoid crimes of violence. [4] Many authorities [5] agree on the frequent sexual outrages, murders

---

[1] Böhmer, *Monatschrift*, p. 206.
[2] Quoted by Böhmer.
[3] Healy, *The Ind. Delinquent*, p. 418 ; Cyril Burt, *The Young Delinquent*, p. 267. Both these authorities admit that there is something in Lombroso's theory, although Burt prefers a new generic term. Gaupp's theory about the connection between dipsomania and epilepsy also points in this direction (Bumke, *Lehrbuch*, p. 650).
[4] Healy, *op. cit.*, p. 423.
[5] Bumke, *Lehrbuch*, pp. 643, 650 ; Viernstein, *Stufenstrafvollzug 3 Bd.*, p. 29 ; Kretschmer, *D. Jur. Zeit.*, p. 785 ; *Med. Psychologie*, p. 222 ; Kretschmer admits that the "insensitive brutal schizoids", "this kind of schizophrenic passion, with its psychological mechanism of a

and other acts of violence by epileptics in their " driven " states. The psychopathological analysis of the epileptoid proportions into " boundness-driven " poles helps us to comprehend the dangers of this temperament.

28. Calm Calculators

Case 34.—Age 19. Supplied ten bottles of wine and a quart of brandy to an Indian. Was with younger boy whom he influenced. Previous convictions for illicit liquor dealing with natives. Unemployed loafer. Pleaded not guilty. In reformatory good blacksmith, but weak scholar. Fond of responsibility, but not a successful leader. Fond of boxing. Extremely fond of a large meal. My observations : usually very calm and phlegmatic, rarely aroused to violent fits of anger, but when aroused he is dangerous ; very calculative and easy-going ; not reliable—no scruples about telling lies when it serves his purpose ; calm self-confidence ; quiet, manly attitude ; dry humour—says if he takes off his boots (for measurements) in this warm weather the doors of the room will have to be opened ; takes a sentence of five years with extreme calmness ; calculative and non-emotional also in his letters. Somatically : Tall, powerful, muscular, athletic (vide Fig. 39).

Many athletics of our material show this type of self-complacent calmness. This boy is so easy-going and phlegmatic, that, in spite of a strong finger, he pulled a weak ergogram in our experiments.[1] It seems as if he could hardly be excited to enthusiasm or strong feelings

latent store of affect, and senseless eruptive outbursts, has many connections with certain brain-traumatic and epileptic syndromes " (*Physique and Character*, p. 170). Vide also Delbrück, *Archiv.* 82, p. 717. Pende, who has studied criminals from an endocrine point of view, says : " In the cynic and blood-thirsty murderers (born criminals) we often find a dyspituitary habitus with signs of a hyper-pituitary-anterior and frequently signs of hypopituitary-posterior " (*Konstitution*, p. 54). This endocrine constellation corresponds exactly to that of the epileptoid athletic both mentally and physically.

[1] Compare with Enke's findings about athletics : uncomplicated, semi-fatalistic attitude ; no apparent affective attitude towards task ; started without saying much ; without hesitation, relatively quick to decide, and matter-of-fact. Skawran (*Typology of Ergograms*), also found that many athletics pulled a weak ergogram. This is especially so when he compared their powerful muscles with their performance. He explains this result as due to their self-confident phlegma (vide Fig. 29b).

of pleasure and emotions which could discharge into his muscles, as in the case of cyclothymes.[1] Neither were there any excitable, timid, self-insufficiency feelings which could urge towards compensatory, strained exertions, as in the leptosomes when pulling ergograms. His phlegmatic disposition is due to complete, manly self-confidence, insusceptibility to emotions generally, and an almost complete absence of sensitivity or excitable timidity.[2] It seems as if the temperament is fully sthenic, without the asthenic " sting " which produces the " hyper-tension and constant offensive against the environment " of the expansive development ; " the purely sthenically experiencing natures are composed and certain in their self-feelings without nervousness, firm and definite also in their most acutely pugnacious acts," says Kretschmer.[3] The gruesome coldness and calmness of the Düsseldorf mass-murderer, Kürten, is also of this kind. These people are very slightly susceptible to any other feelings than self-feelings, and when aroused, to aggressive anger. It is important to bear in mind always that very few, if any of them, are entirely free from violent

[1] Störring emphasizes very strongly the energy contained in the physiological correlates of emotions and feelings (*Psychologie*, p. 216) ; McDougall has shown the connection between emotions and instinctive action (*Social Psychology*) ; and Cannon, too, believes that the Thalamic correlate processes of emotions are sources of energy (*Bodily Changes*, pp. 228, 375). The problem has also been tackled profoundly by physiologists like F. H. Lewy, who reaches the conclusion that autonomic processes and emotions are the main causes of muscular tonus, provided, of course, that well-developed muscles are present (*Vom Lehre der Tonus*, pp. 398, 399, 472, 525, 552). We have also found in experiments with good introspectionists that persons pull a much more convex ergogram when they have worked themselves up emotionally. We believe, however, and shall indicate this in a later chapter, that there are two types of energy, viz. a cortical and sub-cortical one.

[2] Berman says of the prepituitary type : Self-control ; intellectuality ; masculinity ; self-mastery ; calculative ; self-contained ; aggressive sexual hyperactivity (*Glands*, pp. 192, 246, 283). Pende mentions : Logical thinking, masculinity, but also restlessness and irritability (*Konstitution und innere Sekretion*, pp. 22, 36, etc.). Wiessenrieder (*Mitteilungen der Krim. Biol. Gesell.*, 1928, p. 39) describes a typical athletic rational criminal : " The man is a pronounced intellect-centric type ; in spite of strong vegetative, viz. sexual tendencies, he is cool ; in spite of affectivity he is self-controlled." He is strongly self-opinionated.

[3] *Med. Psych.*, 1930, p. 197. Compare v. Wyke case described.

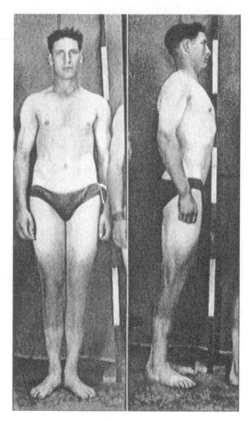

FIG. 39.

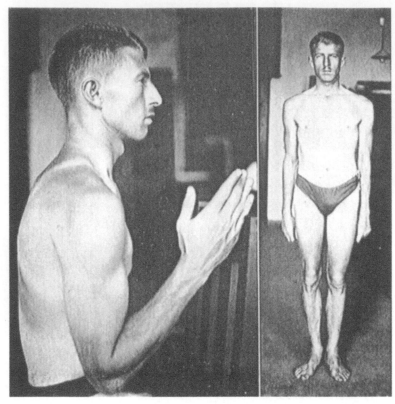

FIG. 40. Athletic with slight Leptosomic strain. Note tetany expression.

aggressiveness at times. In spite of an extremely phlegmatic matrix, crises are bound to develop sometimes (cf. also Case 34). In some of them the manifestations of anger seem purely reactive—a result of provocation. But more usual is one or other inner " drivenness ", hypertension, " black mood," ready to fall on a provoking victim.[1] In some of them the crises are certainly mainly sexually coloured, as in the case of Kürten and the case described by Healy. The crises are probably all connected with pituitary fluctuations.

Together with the phlegma so marked in many athletics, all athletics possess the tendency to perseveration of ideas and aims, in common with the leptosomes (Enke, Pfahler, v. d. Horst, Kretschmer)—or rather, we should say, persistence of intentions (Einstellungen).[2] This quality enables them to construct and premeditate their future acts very planfully, detailedly and systematically. This disposes them not to act impulsively, but in a coldly calculative manner.[3] If it serves their purpose they can organize a mutiny of their fellow-prisoners, only to be able to benefit by reporting it to the authorities, as Kürten did. In our Case No. 36, the juvenile, in order to save his own skin, reported the store-breaking of a native who had served the family faithfully for many years and had broken into the store on the instructions of the lad himself. The young man, described in Case No. 33, would plead energetically for accused boys in the boys' court, only to get them under obligation for his future needs. Their calm self-confidence often jeopardizes their carefulness, so that in some cases of cold scheming by athletics they are not careful enough about subtle details. They are a good combination of calm calculation and careless, broad self-confidence.

---

[1] Cf. with Delbrück's description of these self-controlled epileptoids, who occasionally get into a " driven " state.

[2] We shall still analyse this characteristic psychologically, vide para. 47.

[3] Bumke (*Lehrbuch*, p. 656) mentions that epileptics are very persistent in their obsessions, and may harbour an intention to revenge in a latent state for months and then realize it.

Case 35. Age 19 years. Had a girl in Pretoria ; wanted to be near this girl, and, moreover, felt attracted to the police force generally. Accordingly applied for admittance to police depot in Pretoria. Had no primary school-leaving certificate ; thought about a possible plan ; wrote to a school for his brother's certificate, on which he changed the initials in slightly different ink from the original. Under oath in court still declared that he did not forge certificate. Before this forgery had been discovered, obtained a cheque on request from a dealer, and signed false name in payment for lady's watch, a shirt, socks, braces, soap, cigarettes (total £6).

Father states that boy is beyond control. In reformatory : extremely fond of a big meal ; passion for girls ; very boastful and fond of responsibility ; self-willed ; school-work only done when forced. My finding : typical manner of broad, syrupy, uncritical talking about his own and his relatives' good points ; has been religious throughout his whole life, and comes from a religious stock ; he says none of them has ever worked for the government and nor does he want to. In boys' court very dogmatic, pedantic, and passionate about the infringement of church rules by smaller boys ; speaks with strong conviction. In tests, work, swimming etc., massive and manly self-confidence. Usually very calm and robust self-sufficiency, but occasional driven states, when he is sullen and irritable. Somatically : a tall, powerful athletic—the most burly juvenile at Tokai.

Some of the schemes and calculations of such self-sufficient athletics are indeed very coarse and lack the timid carefulness of leptosomes. Their intrinsic convictions, however, sometimes give much force of persuasion to their explanations. With calm self-confidence and disregard of possible revelations they always try to make the best out of their case in court. They do not confess what is not proved against them. I know an extreme athletic case in South Africa who took careful notes of the evidence. He is so calm and self-confident that in a murder charge against him he laughed when a humourous piece of evidence was given and cross-questioned the witnesses with dramatic ease.[1]

A very remarkable illustration of these bio-psychological

[1] Case v. Wyk. He was executed for this murder.

characteristics is unwittingly given by Professor J. Lange [1] in his studies on the Heufelder identical twins. Adolf is more sly and cunning, uses roundabout ways, prepares and creates his opportunities and defence, denies his guilt until proved, puts the blame on innocent persons to free himself, is cold, defiant, mean and secretive. August, on the other hand, though very similar to Adolf, is less deliberate, takes opportunities when they occur, is frank in his admissions, does not betray his fellows to benefit himself, and is more explosive and uninhibited in court. Lange's photographs indicate that August leans more towards the pyknic physique (his steep, dome-shaped forehead, baldness, round features, shallow eyeballs, straight profile), while Adolf is more athletic (receding forehead, angular profile, athletic chin, elongated egg-shape face).

Leptosomes are also very calculating and secretive; and would desire to free themselves by subterfuges and roundabout ways. But their strong sense of insufficiency and timidity usually seems to counteract the tendency to egotistical exploitation of their fellow beings.

The delinquent act of the boy described in Case No. 34 above, viz. liquor-dealing with natives, is one very frequently found in these non-emotional athletics. We have hardly found a pyknic or a leptosome practising this illicit, but paying, business. One dysplastic athletic explained his illicit liquor-dealing as follows : " It is very simple, sir. I require money, but do not like to do tedious hard work. With liquor-dealing I can make money easily." The person concerned had very few scruples about what his social environment thought of him. Leptosomes, with their sensitivity, striving to compensate, and their ambition on the basis of their fundamental feelings of self-insufficiency and timidity, usually care very consciously what the environment thinks of them. It is the old

---

[1] Professor J. Lange, *Verbrechen als Schicksal*, Leipsig, 1929, p. 24. In some of the other twins described by Lange, Kretschmer's typology can also be applied.

antithesis : I and the external world ; a constant, excited self-analysis and comparison, as Kretschmer says. Pyknics are much more naive and do not reflect about the self. But still, pyknics form such an easy, frank, natural integration with the environment, are so apt to emotionally identify themselves with their fellow-beings, that they cannot seriously diverge from the views and social valuations of their environment. Pyknics retain the inner rapport and consensus with their environment. If we analyse these cases of athletics carefully, we find neither the timid, sensitive striving for "assurances" of the leptosome, nor the natural inner rapport of the pyknic. Athletics are self-contained, self-confident, and egocentric.[1] The innate conviction which accompanies every act and judgment of them renders them immune to the critical attitude of others and, as Delbrück says, incapable of auto-criticism.[2] Thinking and acting, intelligence and impulse-life, is a too narrowly coherent unity (Delbrück). The result is immunity to heterocentric contradictions, lack of social scruples.

In normal and intellectual athletics this quality may be extremely valuable ; the athletic Haeckel was able to face the world with his doctrines of evolution and monistic materialism.[3] But in crime this quality may take the form of a degenerated form of egotism and almost complete absence of scruples about what society thinks, or absence of fear for social deprecation, ostracism, etc. The dysplastic athletic mentioned above lived together with a coloured woman in concubinage for a considerable time—an act extremely loathed by white South Africans.

The absence of social scruples is not the only psychological cause of illicit liquor-dealing with natives. Athletics are prone to this crime for some or all of the following reasons :—

---

[1] Berman, *Glands Regulating Personality*, pp. 246 and 247. Delbrück, *Archiv. f. Psych. und Nervenkrankh.*, 1928, p. 714.

[2] Delbrück, *op. cit.*, p. 717.

[3] Haeckel, Ernst, *The Riddle of the Universe*, etc. Haeckel was probably a more undaunted fighter for Darwinism than Darwin himself.

(*a*) They are frequently addicted to drink, themselves, and as such are in the liquor atmosphere and know how and where to purchase liquor without danger of suspicion or detection.

(*b*) They are able to bargain manfully with the buyers.

(*c*) The calm calculativeness of this type of athletic aids him in the execution of this netherworld business.

(*d*) Their egocentric lack of scruples about the social deprecation and lack of conscientious sympathy with the primitive races whom they ruin in this way, add to the motivation value of their calm calculations on the profitableness of the practice. One athletic of our material had a bicycle with a bag between the frame rods. Saturdays were his delivering days, when he took bags of bottles with brandy to the coloured buyers. These bottles he bought from various bottle stores, and spread over all the other days of the week in order to prevent suspicion.

29. *Boasters and Swindlers*

Bumke speaks about the " broad, complacent philosophizing about themselves " in the talk of epileptic personalities.

They deem themselves better than all others. These extremes in the clinical material have their corresponding normal characterological forms, and in some delinquents this characteristic again takes on grotesque proportions. We have not had enough such cases in our material to judge definitely whether these qualities derive more frequently from epileptoid or from hypomanic self-feelings, and in how far they are connected with " pseudologia phantastica ".[1]

---

[1] In a supreme court case a few months ago, such an outspoken athletic told tales about buried money, etc., which certainly points in the direction of pseudologia. He speaks with such an inner conviction that the court even believed him and released him. (In the meantime in a second murder trial this man, v. Wyk, tried the same remarkably " convincing " stories about thousands of buried pounds. He was allowed to search for them under escort. Previous to this he had duped many moneylenders with similar tales. Pseudologists in Kronfeld's sense they certainly are. Cf. Schneider, *Psychopath. Pers.*, p. 58; Bumke, *Lehrbuch*, p. 270 ; Healy, *op. cit.*, p. 427.)

The most pronounced cases were athletics with slight pyknic admixture.

Case 36.—Age 20 years. Stole second-hand guns from a storeroom ; got his native servant to bury them in his hut and to try and sell them to natives in Basutoland for oxen. Natives would not buy guns without ammunition, so he persuaded his two native servants to break into a store where ammunition was sold. He indicated to them how to enter through the skylight. The natives were unable to get the ammunition, and thereupon he reported them to the storekeeper, stating that he could put him on the track for a reward of £50.

Sold liquor to natives by leaving bottles in his workshop and paid his native servant one bottle for every four bottles that he sold. In court he stated that he drank heavily, and that the liquor had been stolen from him by the natives. Previous convictions : common theft at the age of 16 ; assault at the age of 18, and again shortly before committal. Very fond of speculation with crude methods. In reformatory: intellectual and practical abilities, but very lazy and easy-going ; boastful. My observations : Extremely fond of talking about himself, his past, and especially about his business transactions which were successful. States he wanted to get rich quickly. Had the contract for gravelling the streets ; owned a plumber's shop with nine registered workmen under him ; at the same time wild stock speculations ; bought 300 oxen in Rhodesia and sold them at tremendous profits in the Union ; stole 200 guns from Government and bartered cattle with these ; swam full river to get into Basutoland in order to barter ; speaks, reads and writes two native languages; possesses many hundreds of pounds in cash as well as a fine motor car, but was not allowed to pay a fine for crimes. (As far as I could ascertain, most of these statements are untrue.) Hardly ever laughs, but with a self-complacent smile and sparkling eyes he tells all these stories. He has no scruples whatsoever, and says so himself. Drank heavily in pre-reformatory days and misbehaved himself promiscuously with all types of girls indiscriminately. Does not want to work in reformatory, he declares, because not paid for it. He is extremely calm and easy-going: does not partake in sport or swimming. Very fond of a heavy meal.

In general life we have also frequently met with such boasters with primarily athletic constitution. They can even be differentiated from pyknic hypomanic boasters. These athletics boast for two reasons : First, to mislead women or creditors from whom they are to receive. Secondly, they talk and moralize with broad complacence about their own virtues and sacrifices in conformity with the intrinsic self-sufficiency and egocentricity of epileptoids [1] (vide Case 35).

With their pedantic ego-centricity these athletics seem to be incapable of real self-criticism, sense of self-insufficiency, on the basis of careful introspection : " An epileptoid will never be able to scrutinize himself critically," says Delbrück.[2] The inward directedness of attention (Autism) is not common to athletics. A student of Jaensch found in his disintegrated athletics and sportsmen that they were disinclined to self-observation.[3] In daily life we have also ascertained from athletics that, though they may be persistently occupied with an objective problem, they very rarely scrutinize their own subjective motives and convictions critically. That is why athletics are susceptible to " broad, complacent speculations about the self ", even to the extremes of boasting and swindling, unaccompanied by " subjective inhibitions ". Their narrow viewpoints and intolerant rigorism also derives largely from this lack of hetero-centricity. Such egocentric ideas are easily accompanied by the firmly rooted consciousness of validity. The contradictory ideas connected with feelings of self-insufficiency are derivatively inhibited from their narrow consciousness.[4] As is explained

---

[1] Kronfeld (quoted by Schneider, *op. cit.*, p. 58) distinguishes between phantast and pseudologist. The former dupes himself, the latter dupes the environment. Our athletics seem to be more inclined towards pseudologism in this sense, although phantasticism is also present to some extent. We see here how near the epileptoid's uncritical verbosity is to hysterical vanity ; both have the factors of self-assertion (Geltungsucht).

[2] Delbrück, *Archiv.* 82, p. 717.

[3] Möckelmann, *Personlichkeitstypus des Turners und Sportlers*, Marburg, 1921, p. 35.

[4] Strong convictions accompany every act and judgment of the epileptoid, according to Delbrück. We can understand how feelings of self-confidence and activity can derivatively inhibit from consciousness all other feelings of insecurity (Störring). The result will be that only ideas conforming to the self-confident frame of mind are allowed in

by Birnbaum, the lack of self-critical uncertainty adds tremendously to the persuasive powers of a swindler. They are universally believed and trusted on the basis of their self-certainty.

The lack of critical self-scrutiny described is intimately connected with the essential characteristics of the " masterful leaders " and aggressive types of athletics described previously. Leptosomes are characterized by self-insufficient retiring to a sensitive self-life (Autism), athletics by a too narrow connection between ideational systems and motorical execution, without the inhibitions of hetero-centricity and critical self-scrutiny.[1]

30. Alcoholism

Alcoholism is mentioned by Kretschmer as an important ingredient of the epileptoid syndrome.[2] Delbrück gives a typical example of a dipsomanic tendency in an epileptoid mathematics teacher. Gaupp defines dipsomania as : " spasmodic appearance of characteristic conditions, when, after preceding ill-humour, an irresistible impulse is experienced towards indulgence in intoxicating drink and towards great excesses, accompanied by, or gradually leading up to, a slighter or deeper clouding of consciousness, until after a few hours or days, occasionally after months, the attack ends spontaneously and after the intoxicants have been worked off makes place for more or less normal conditions." In this form Gaupp took dipsomania as a purely epileptic symptom.[3] Bumke acknowledges the frequent appearance of dipsomania in the epileptic syndrome but does not take it as exclusively epileptoid. Healy also mentions the connection between dipsomanic attacks and the tall muscular body-build.[4]

consciousness, and conflicting ideas connected with feelings of insecurity are inhibited (Störring, *Psch.*, p. 200).

[1] Delbrück says : " Narrowly, too narrowly connected are impulse-life, emotions and intelligence." The intelligence and impulse-life (movements), especially, are extremely intimately connected. They think in movements, so to speak.

[2] Kretschmer, *Deutsche. Jur. Zeit.* 31, p. 785; *Med. Psych.*, p. 222.

[3] Bumke, *Lehrbuch*, p. 650.

[4] Healy, *The Indiv. Delinquent*, p. 429.

Our own material is too limited to permit definite conclusions. We may give the following observations in regard to our material. Very few athletics above the age of 18 years are entirely free from addiction to intoxicants.[1] As already stated, many of them practice illicit liquor-dealing with natives. Athletics, however, are not the only alcoholic delinquents. As Bumke and Kretschmer mention, hypomanic cyclothymes also tend to alcoholic excesses. It is possible that the flowing transitions between the hypomanic cyclothyme and the athletic temperament has some connection with this. But it is probable that in typical cases cyclothymic drinkers show more sensual, comfortable enjoyment, while athletics show more blind drivenness in their drinking. In both types the desire to play the hero has much to do with their dipsomanic ruses.

31. *Sexuality*

With the more plump dysplastic athletic we shall still deal separately. The tall athletics of our material do not seem to have so many sexual difficulties as leptosomes. Two very powerfully built athletics (Cases 33 and 34) pretended to us during the interview that they have a disinclination to sexual relations with women. Both of them were observed, however, to be fond of dirty sex talk and pictures of nude women. The father of Case No. 34 was also a tall athletic and had sixteen children. We very often found in private life, and also in the families of our delinquent material, that large families are typical for athletics. From Cases 36 and 35, and 28, which are typical, it is obvious that athletic boys above the age of 18 are inclined to promiscuous behaviour; and it is fairly definite in our material, that in their sexual relations athletics are very little influenced by erotic idealism. The bare physical relations, in many cases indiscriminately

---

[1] Some were even addicted to Dagga-smoking—a South African herb (*Cannabis indicus*) with particularly clouding influences on consciousness and heightening of self-feelings.

with all kinds of women, are the central aims.[1] The Düsseldorf murderer, Kürten, apart from sadistic perversions, had a strong physical sexuality which must even have been a hereditary taint, because Kürten's father had been convicted of sexual relations with servant girls. Healy also mentions that strong sexuality is correlated with epilepsy, and that the strongest sex impulse he met in his whole psychiatric career, was an athletic epileptoid.[2]

It is not yet certain whether the manifestations of physical sexuality of athletics in the form of promiscuous misbehaviour or excessive intercourse with their own wives [3] are due to a strong sexual impulse, or to the absence of inhibitions (such as self-critical insufficiency, lack of tender consideration for women, and of idealistic eroticism, etc.). As far as our experience goes, we are inclined to believe that both factors are involved.

The athletic constitution seems to be the normal masculinistic one.[4] We should, therefore, expect a strong development of the male sexuality in this habitus. We shall see, in a later chapter, that the athletic habitus has very close relationships with the anterior pituitary gland and its neural controls. Most authorities [5] on endocrinology agree that insufficient pituitary secretion goes with sexual retardatoin and hyperpituitarism favours hypersexuality in the male. It becomes more and more probable that migraine, some epileptic fits, spasmodic sexual ruses, dipsomania, and epileptoid crises of aggressive-

---

[1] Berman says (*op. cit.*, p. 270): "This explosive periodicity of the sexual life (as in Napoleon) with a tendency to compression of its expression to the merely physical is another mark of some pituitary-centred personalities." I have frequently noticed that, though pyknics and leptosomes are usually attracted to one another in marriage, athletics usually marry with athletics, perhaps because athletics are physically attracted to one another.

[2] *The Ind. Delinquent*, p. 427.

[3] I know an athletic in private life, who had sexual intercourse regularly with his wife at least three times a night. He could hardly abstain during her menstrual indispositions. The woman died in childbirth (her tenth one) at the age of 37.

[4] Berman, pp. 196, 243; Pende, p. 13.

[5] Kuntz, *Autonomic Nervous System*, Philadelphia, 1929; Berman, *op. cit.*; Pende, etc.

ness, are all related to fluctuations in anterior-pituitary, neuroglandular functions.[1] It is possible that extreme functions of this gland, as is found in acromegaly, may again act antagonistically on the sexuality.

32. Tensions in Athletics

It is possible to understand theoretically, how any neural and neuroglandular excitement is transformed into a strong dynamic moment (hypertensions) in the athletic constitution. The school of Jaensch,[2] have found that in sportsmen of the T-type, the functional significance of kinaesthetic images and sensations is very pronounced. We may construe it in this way, that, while the average adult thinks and imagines primarily in terms of visual images, verbal representations, etc.; well-trained athletics represent (vorstellen) their images, ideas and intentions mainly by kinaesthetic images, supported by slight, reproduced ("tentative") movements,[3] i.e. they actually act their thoughts, or think and imagine in movements. In athletics, therefore the connections between thinking and imagining on the one hand, and motor processes on the other, are extremely intimate. These connections become narrower with frequent use of the motor-system.[4] The affinity between the athletic constitution and epilepsy is another point of evidence in favour of the athletic's susceptible motor regions; because motor excitability is a primary characteristic of epileptics.[5]

The investigations of F. H. Lewy[6] and others, make it seem probable that the tonus, or static (postural) innervation

---

[1] Berman, pp. 283, 276, 244.

[2] Möckelmann, op. cit., p. 14.

[3] Recent investigations appear to indicate that in all human beings thinking-processes are accompanied or supported by "tentative" movements (Washburn in "Feelings and Emotions", Wittenberg Symposium, Clark Univ., 1928, p. 105). In athletics the motor side would then only be more accentuated than in the average case.

[4] W. Jaensch, Grundzüge, p. 79.

[5] Störring, Psychologie, p. 195; Bumke, Lehrbuch, p. 642; Kreyenberg, op. cit., p. 592. Jaensch, Grundzüge, p. 276.

[6] F. H. Lewy, Die Lehre vom Tonus und der Bewegung, Berlin, 1923, p. 81.

of the hard skeletal muscles of athletics must be very good, because the tonus of the muscle, when at rest, can be fairly well gauged from its hardness. This state of tonus, according to Lewy, Kuntz, etc., depends largely on

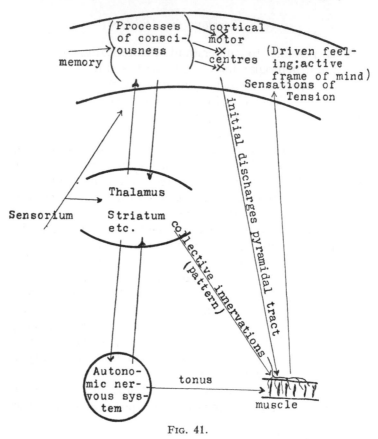

FIG. 41.

endocrine and autonomic (vagus and sympathetic) functions.[1] The works of Pende, Berman, Cannon, etc., seem to show that well-toned skeletal musculature depends upon the adrenal (particularly the cortex) glands, and their sub-cortical (thalamo-striate) neural controls. The

[1] F. H. Lewy, *op. cit.* ; Kuntz, *The Autonomic Nervous System*, Philadelphia, 1929.

tonus conceived in this way, is a rest (static, postural) state to be distinctly kept apart from cerebro-spinal movement (dynamic) innervations. The external movement of a limb, therefore, depends on two factors : the tonus (static innervation, or preparedness) and cerebrospinal (voluntary, dynamic, or alterative) innervations. The tonus seems to be largely a sub-cortical (thalamostriate) and autonomic function, while the voluntary innervation is a cortical (pyramidal) function.[1] But the position is not so simple as it seems. Even if the tonus is a sub-cortical function, feelings and emotions are certainly very intimately connected with the tonus, the thalamostriate brain and the autonomic (vegetative) nervous system on the one hand, and cortical processes (correlates of ideas, images, sensations, etc.), on the other hand. Cortical processes may, therefore, by way of emotions and feelings, influence the tonus.[2] But apart from such influences on tonus, via the thalamo-striate centres, and the vegetative system, cortical processes appear to influence directly the static innervation or tension state of the muscles prior to the actual movement. Prior to the external movement, the muscles are tensioned by slight initial discharges of nerve-energy along the pyramidal nerves, and by collective (pattern) innervations from the thalamostriatum under cortical control. This state of tension (due to initial discharges) before the actual external movement takes place (Störring), is also described by Lewy as " Sperrung ".[3] The tonus of muscles, therefore, though also connected with the thalamo-striate centres and emotions, etc., is largely a function of the vegetative nervous system. Tension, or Sperrung, on the other hand, presupposes cortical innervation, or cortical control, though here, too, sub-cortical processes (Cannon) and emotions, excitement (Störring) are co-involved (mitbeteiligt). According to Störring this muscular tension—as distinguished from muscular tonus—gives rise to sensations

---

[1] Lewy, *op. cit.*, pp. 399, 466, 474, 513 ; Kuntz, *op. cit.* ; W. Jaensch, *Grundzüge*, p. 296, 300, 306.

[2] Cf. also, Lewy, p. 553.

[3] Lewy, *op. cit.*, pp. 513–5 ; Störring, *Psychologie*, pp. 221, 223, 225.

of tension and active frames of mind (vide Fig. 41).[1] But tonus is certainly also involved in the production of sensations of tension. First, the tension (Sperrung), i.e. the result of initial innervations depends largely on the tonus of the muscle ; the initial discharges will have much less effect on atonic muscles than on the well-toned muscles of athletics. Secondly, we submit that Störring's theory must be so modified that any tonic or tensioned state of the musculature, be it autonomically, sub-cortically, or cortically induced, provided that this tonus or tension is sufficiently intense, gives rise to sensations of tension, active frames of mind, motor-urge, or "driven" feelings (vide Fig. 41). It is possible that in this respect later research may find differences in the nature of tensions in different constitution-types. At the present stage of research, the whole problem concerning the exact nature of discharges (into the musculature) of nervous energy, connected with mental processes is far from solved ; Störring thinks the mental energy discharges via the cortical motor-centres, while Cannon seems to accept that the thalamus is the source of emotional energy, whence (under cortical control) it is directly discharged downwards.[2] Most modern authorities (Störring, Cannon, McDougall, Bumke, etc.), however, seem to agree that mental processes, particularly emotions and feelings, are connected with nervous energy, which in some form or other, discharges into the musculature to produce changes of tonus, and, in co-operation with, or via the cortical motor-centres, also muscular tensions (initial innervations) and actual overt movement. Particularly in athletics, who, as a type, have the most susceptible motor-system and the best-toned muscles, any nervous discharges will produce prompt and strong increase of tonus and tension in the muscles with resultant consciousness of tension, active frame of mind, and " drivenness ". Such nervous

---

[1] Störring, op. cit., p. 223. This tension-state has much in common with Washburn's " activity attitude " and " tentative movements " (Feelings and Emotions, Clark Univ., 1928, p. 105).

[2] According to Cannon's theory and evidence the "felt" urge or " drivenness " may be due to impulses from the thalamus upwards.

discharges are connected with all neural and neuro-glandular upheavals (emotions, excitement, etc.). Fluctuations in the pituitary functions, *sella turcica* troubles, reactive anger, sexual waves, etc., may all of them initiate or constitute charges of nervous energy, ready to flow over into the well-toned and susceptible musculature.

Although the detailed mechanisms must still be worked out, at the present stage of research it seems probable, therefore, that psychical tensions, states of " drivenness " and active frames of mind, as they appear in epileptoid crises, depend on two main factors : on well-toned, large muscles, and on neural and neuro-glandular excitement.

SUMMARY OF CONCLUSIONS

1. Clinical studies appear to indicate a biological affinity between the athletic constitution and the epileptic syndrome. The epileptoid polarity " Driven-bound " as analysed by Delbrück is a plausible working hypothesis.

2. The two poles may be in co-function as in systematic and persistently aggressive persons.

3. The " Driven " crises which develop on the calm matrix of the athletic temperament, explain the very frequent aggressive violence of athletic delinquents.

4. The manly self-confidence of athletics disposes them to undaunted criminal acts, and disregard of social deprecation.

5. Egocentricity, lack of fear and of social scruples, " driven " crises, calculativeness, etc., make athletic criminals very dangerous and of a weak social prognosis.

6. Calm, unscrupulous calculativeness (as a calm matrix on which crises may develop) is very pronounced in the athletic delinquents. This phlegma is also manifested in the ergograms of many athletics.

7. In their " bound "-pole athletics are inclined to a broad self-complacent speculation about their own super-qualities. This may degenerate into a type of pseudology.

8. Alcoholic and sexual ruses are intimately related to the driven crises, and all these mental manifestations are probably connected with pituitary functions.

9. The " drivenness " and tensions which are such important factors in the epileptoid mind, can be explained according to the scheme given.

CHAPTER VI

MENTAL QUALITIES (INCLUDING DELINQUENCY) OF PYKNICS

33. *Cyclothymy*

Even Bumke who believes that schizothymy is an ingenious, but nevertheless artificial construction, accepts the cyclothyme temperament as a valid constitutional type, differing from the constitutional mental disease of manic-depression by degrees only and showing a biological affinity to the pyknic habitus.[1] We may rest assured that cyclothymy and its biological connections with the pyknic habitus is accepted by almost all modern psychiatrists.

The cyclothyme temperament has also a polarity, a range of proportions, like the bound-driven proportions of the epileptoid and the sensitive-cold proportions of the schizothyme, The diathetic proportions of the cyclothymes correspond to the psychotic extremes of mania and depression. Kretschmer gives them as :—

" Cheerful, humorous, jolly, hasty "

for the mania side, and :—

" Quiet, calm, easily depressed, soft-hearted "

for the depression side.

In addition to these proportions he gives the fundamental marks of the cyclo-temperament as " Sociable, good-natured, friendly, genial ".

If we compare all these qualities of the cyclo-temperament with the epilepto- or the schizo-temperament, it is obvious that the latter two are socially much less desirable

---

[1] Bumke, *Lehrbuch*, pp. 327, 204, 208, 687, 758 ; Delbrück, *op. cit.*, p. 714, puts forth the argument that if a somatic correlation is possible in cyclothymy, it encourages us at least to look for one in schizothymy and epileptoidy.

than the first-mentioned.   To a large extent we shall find this fact verified in everyday life and in insusceptibility to serious criminality.   But, as already mentioned,[1] Kretschmer seems to favour the cyclothymes unduly.   We shall see that, especially under the hypomaniacs, we find many undesirables (such as self-feeling querulants, lazy enjoyers, etc.) who are smoothed over in Kretschmer's depictions.

The diathetic proportions of exalted-depressed may in some individuals be more marked at the exalted pole (the hypomaniacs).   In other individuals, as Kretschmer indicates, the exaltation and depression may alternate in successive periods of various durations, or, as Thalbitzer maintains, the exaltation-depression may be present simultaneously, but with reference to different aims or objects.[2]   In still another group the depressive pole dominates.   In our own material we have hardly found a single pure depressive.   But we shall shortly refer to some cases described by other investigators.   The maniac pole of the cyclo's seems to be, both somatically and psychically, nearest the athletic's which we have discussed. Therefore, we can conveniently start our exposition at the extreme manic pole.   We may here again refer to our *Triangle of Temperaments* (para. 58) for a clear conception of the gradual transitions from athletics over hypomanic pyknics, to depressed pyknics, and from these to leptosomes again.   In a special chapter on the physiological bases of these types we shall endeavour to show that such a scheme can be supported by many facts in neuroglandular researches.   These interpretations are, however, at the present stage of research, very tentative, but could nevertheless serve as a working scheme to be modified and completed by later researches.

34.   *Masters and Bullies ; Querulants ; Choleric, Aggressive Self-feelings ; Impatient, Fiery Temperaments*

Case 37.—Age 17½ years.   Bought following articles in the names of grandmother and aunt with whom he had resided

---

[1] Pfahler, *System der Typenlehren*, p. 169.
[2] Thalbitzer, *Emotion and Insanity*, London, 1926.

for ten years previous to his going into employment two years ago : ladies' fawn fur, £1 10s. ; ladies' shoes, 8s. 6d. ; gents' shoes, hose, ties, shirts, blazer, and razor outfit, total, £8. Hired car under false pretensions and drove 127 miles with it, returning after midnight. His father, also short and stoutly built, had had trouble with his mother and was divorced. Boy wayward and gives much trouble as a disobedient, aggressive, quarrelsome child. Frequently changed work, because fickle and quarrelsome. Previously convicted for fraud on three occasions. Very cruel to animals when younger.

My observations : Terrific, sullen self-assertions, repeatedly asked me and teachers to get into a gaol where hard work and iron bars could isolate him from the distracting outside world. He detests the interference of reformative officers, and the provocative semi-freedom of the reformatory : says he has definitely decided to revenge himself in some way or other and escape by violence. Sexual extravagances in free life ; will never be tamed, he says, as long as there are girls, motor-cars, etc., because he wants what he sees ; fond of aeroplanes and adventure.

Somatically well-built pyknic ; peculiar feature being heavy fat-accumulation on buttocks (compare with dysplastic cases 60 and 61).

Case 38.—Age 18 years. Two convictions for house-breaking and theft ; one for theft of motor-cycle. Committed to reformatory because repeatedly absconded from reformative hostel, where he was certified incorrigible.

My observations: Self-assertive type, unsympathetic expression ; fairly restless during interview ; fond of sports, quick-tempered with fellows ; obstinate self-feelings in letters ; very self-willed and strongly refractory to forceful interference, e.g. in religion, parental control, etc. Somatically a pyknic with athletic admixture such as long legs (vide Fig. 44.)

Case 39.—Letter written to his mother by a well-built pyknic of 18 years : " Dear mother, Just a few lines to let you know that I am still quite well, hoping to hear the same from you. Mother, you must give me a job somewhere, it is high time that I have left this school and started work. You must answer my letters in future, and let me know how you are going on. I always let you know how I am getting on, but you don't think of letting me know anything. You know as I feel as if I could shoot myself this moment the way you treat me. A person would think I was a dog the way you carry on with me. I am going to try to find a job myself and if I do get one I will go my own way. None of you must try and stop me because that one will have to stand the consequences. Before I give a penny away I will drink it out the same as my own dear father did. I know that you often think that I can go to hell for your part and I will too. You need not get me a work if you don't want to. I am not hard up for your money. I will earn my own one day and then I can do as I like with it, drink it out or waist it in some other way if I like. That Mr. C. (his stepfather) thinks he has a big son that can work for him one day, but he is very mistaken. I would see him in the hot world before I would give him a farthing. I am going to start Goozen's (a notorious criminal) stunts one day and then we will see who can be boss, me or the rest of the family.

I remain your haited son . . .—

P.S.—Now you will feel what it is when your son is sitting in hell. Give this letter to that Mr. C. You brought me into this world and this is what you do to me now, leaving me to find my own way in this old world.

You must not get a fright one day when you get the tiding that I have shot myself. It may be this year."

This boy is very boastful and naively assuming, even towards his teachers. On his release from the institution, he went to his father, quarrelled with him and his step-mother very disrespectfully, squandered his money, could not stay in any employment. His brother is very much the same build and temperament, and his father (same build) has been repeatedly convicted of assault.

Thalbitzer says : " This expansive anger is so usual in mania, that it really belongs to the standard type of mania ".[1] In his analysis of this variant of mania, Thalbitzer shows that it is a mixture of unpleasure directed on some object, and pleasure connected with " the idea of the angry man himself and his position as the person who is in the right and who, therefore, can think himself as the superior party perhaps punishing and chastising." This self-feeling is certainly the main spindle around which everything revolves. The following characterization—according to Thalbitzer, reminiscent of mania—is essentially true of our cases : " Bad-humoured, peevish, argumentative, self-opinionated patient with

[1] Thalbitzer, *Emotion and Insanity*, p. 63.

his delight in contradiction and criticism and his inclination to annoy, irritate, and plague those around him." Bumke also mentions these hypomaniac querulants, as "professional brawlers" and "quarrelsome scolds".[1] They seem to form flowing transitions between the hypomanic disposition and the paranoid querulants.[2] These transitional types are not so much paranoid querulants as what Klug[3] calls "situation-querulants". The theme or situation about which they quarrel is a new one every time. They resemble the child between the ages of 2 and 4 years who bumps with his aimless willing and strong, naïve self-feelings against numerous and varied limitations imposed by the environment. The hypomanic querulants have the high, naïve self-feelings and the lively activity of the hypomanic disposition, but they may also reveal an additional (epileptoid ?) characteristic usually not found in the typical hypomanics : they are to a large extent incapable of respecting the feelings of others. This is in conformance with Kretschmer's contention that such querulatoric cyclothymes are constitutionally mixed. Our own cases show athletic and dysplastic admixture (vide para. 44). In private life we have met such a "professional quarreller" who suffers from dipsomanic crises and reveals himself to his neighbours as a loud, overbearing disputer. He has a real pyknic body, fat belly, short neck, broad lower face, but with the following admixture : Broad shoulders, fair muscles, heavy long eyebrows, and a medium skull circumference which makes his head slightly towering from the thick neck and fat from lower face upwards.[4] They seem to be pyknics with a fair amount of athletic-dysplastic admixture (refer also Cases 60, 61).

But these cases are so near the manic group that they

---

[1] Bumke, *Grenzen der Geistigen Gesundheit*, p. 12 ; *Lehrbuch*, pp. 203, 328, 342 ; Kretschmer, *Physique and Character*, p. 136.

[2] Bumke, *Lehrbuch*, pp. 367, 340, 205 ; *Grenzen, etc.*, p. 12. Vide also Kretschmer, *Med. Psych.*, p. 195.

[3] *Stufenstrafvollzug* (1929), p. 111. Vide also K. Schneider, *op. cit.*, p. 31.

[4] This case, however, was also very conscious of a physical defect (rupture) which may have much to do with the temperament. Bumke, *Lehrbuch*, 206, 342.

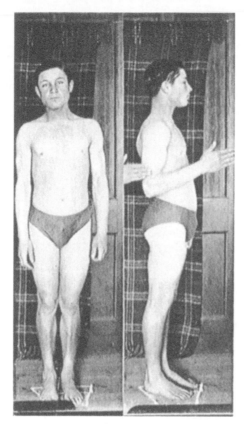

FIG. 42.

[*face p.* 180

should be classified under the cyclothymes. Most of them are, as Kretschmer says of the pyknic, hypomanic aggressives, "relatively harmless," "tractable by means of humour," "constitutionally sociable."[1] In fact, in some of these the aggressive crises form isolated reactions in an otherwise attractive behaviour. Such aggressive crises are then usually due to sufficient provocation. They are stimulus-adequate, aggressive reactions in a wave-form. In these reactive crises, as well as in the more querulatoric hypomanic attitudes, in fact, in all cyclothymic behaviour, the following characterizations by Kretschmer are admirably illustrated : "lack of system," "poverty of systematic construction," "lack of inhibitions," "fiery temperament," "well rounded, wavelike, natural responses," "when anything gets in his way he sees red at once," "cannot swallow his indignation . . . for that reason he bears no malice," brooding intrigue and deferred revenge are foreign to him.[2] It is in this respect that the typical hypomanic cyclothyme differs from the epileptoid who, according to Bumke, resorts to knives even when the provocation lies many months in the past.[3] The cyclothyme flares up suddenly, makes an impulsive row to attain his end, and is soon pacified. These impulsive rows may take on very drastic forms, however, and are a hypomanic characteristic which figures very largely in studies on criminals.[4] The following cases give some idea

---

[1] *Deutsche Jur. Zeit.*, 31, p. 785.

[2] We can compare the cyclothyme temperamentally with early childhood. All the characteristics mentioned above remind one of the child's first wilfulness (Erstes Trotzalter of Ch. Bühler's *Seelenleben des Jugendlichen*, pp. 45, 104). The child begins to will without having a definite aim to will, therefore Ch. Bühler calls it "purely formal aimless willing"; of the child's quarrelsome self-feelings at the age of 2 to 3 years : "A strong anti-social wave overcomes the three-year-old. He can be inimical towards everybody. His strong stirring will knocks against limits in all directions." (Vide also K. Bühler, *Die Geistige Entwicklung des Kindes*, Jena, 1930, p. 129).

[3] Bumke, *Lehrbuch*, p. 656. This is probably due to a persistence of Einstellung, or what Pfahler would term perseveration. "Perseveration" of intentions or attitudes plays a much smaller rôle in the cyclothymes.

[4] This hypomanic explosive anger is very well known in studies on criminals. Compare Kretschmer, *op. cit.*, 31, p. 785. Klug,

of what may happen in a delinquent cyclothyme, when he rocks out of his customary, comfortable enjoyment, or jovial, naïve self-feelings into an aggressive reaction on provocation, and then back to normality :—

Case 40.—Age 19 years. Convicted of culpable homicide on his father. Father a heavy drinker, wasted two farms in this way. Boy, eldest child, tried to keep finances going ; reported his father's drunkenness to his grandfather ; this annoyed father ; grandfather presented father with a new farm on condition that the drinking should stop ; father submitted to this for some months ; then suddenly exchanged his whole wool-clip for drink ; he arrived home heavily intoxicated, quarrelled with sister of convicted who thereupon threatened that he would again tell his grandfather; boy went to his room to get possession of gun because on previous intoxications father had fired on natives, etc. ; father called boy, the latter refused to come, and instead threatened to shoot his father if he came nearer to him. Father approached, dressed in his shirt only; boy became very angry, shot father through stomach. On seeing father drop to the ground he felt very sorry, prayed in his room that father might be spared, reported himself to police, stating that he did not know what he did when he pulled the trigger.

In reformatory : violent waves of anger when sufficiently provoked, otherwise a pleasant, sociable, humorous disposition ; excellent work in blacksmith's shop and school ; good prognosis ; frank and manly, matter-of-fact attitude in tests ; humorous recitals in boys' debates ; very easy and frank in measurements and photographs ; affective letters to his home ; heartfelt religion ; given to mischief-making ; liked by the boys for his gift of mimicry ; fond of girls, smoking and swearing ; generous towards fellows. Somatically : pyknic, but with fair amount of muscles on shoulders, arms and legs.

Case 41.—Age 13 years. Stole 2s. from a fellow in an orphanage. Repeated attempts to escape from the orphanage, escaped three times from previous house of refuge. Previously stole two tins of jam from a store ; smokes large quantities

---

Stufenstrafvollzug (1929), p. 93 ; Viernstein, *Stufenstrafvollzug* (1929), p. 29 ; Pende, *op. cit.*, p. 8 ; K. Schneider, *Psychopath. Personl.*, p. 32. In normal psychology Enke has found very impatient and quickly angered (*op. cit.*, pp. 263, 267). Jaensch maintains the same of his B-type (*Grundzüge*, p. 165). Lenz, *Grundriss der Krim. Biol.*, 1927, pp. 177, 189.

of cigarettes when obtainable, stealing money to buy these. When locked up for misbehaviour, he became vicious, tried to force door, had to be guarded night and day until police took charge of him. In reformatory received fifty-nine cuts during a period of three years, mostly for excessive smoking, false statements, disrespect, and theft. During investigation, showed discontent as if unwilling to be tested, but afterwards became more sociable. Is very easy-going, and the type that will rather smoke in comfort, shirk from work, and show gross insolence when provoked, than try conscientiously to earn badges.

Somatically : pyknic, but fairly long nose and fair musculature, indicating athletic admixture (vide Fig. 42).

The first case, in his normal periods, shows the pleasant, sociable, generous, and active disposition which, according to Kretschmer, is much more frequent than the melancholic variant of cyclothymy. But when his environment provokes him, "he sees red," he gets blind with anger and reacts impulsively. Immediately after he regrets his act, shows real sympathy, and tries his utmost to correct his misdeeds.[1] One of our " fiery temperaments " was an easy, sociable juvenile who, on request, described to me many of the temperaments of his fellows in a witty and masterful manner. With remarkable, calm boldness, he stole food for his starving mother. But on certain occasions when she provoked him, he swung into violent states of anger and fired several shots at her with his revolver.[2] He remembered very little about these, when the storm was over, and he then assumed his former kindly relations with her.

The second case given above belongs to the " comfortable

[1] Compare with Bumke's descriptions of the hypomanics, *Lehrbuch,* p. 203 ; also *Stufenstrafvollzug* (1929), pp. 29, 93.

[2] It is important to note here that McDougall (*National Welfare and National Decay,* pp. 96, 109) mentions the frequency of crimes of violence —especially homicide—among the southern peoples of Europe. We know definitely that pyknics are more frequent in the southern than in the northern races (compare also E. R. and W. Jaensch's investigations). McDougall explains the frequency of homicide instead of suicide, on the basis of the racial characteristics of the south, " vivacious, quick, impetuous, and impulsive, their emotions blaze out vividly and instantaneously into violent expression and action." McDougall, with some hesitation, proposes that the southern races are more prone to force than to divorce as a means of solving marital infidelity problems.

enjoyers " in normal times (jam, smoking, laziness). When treated with force, he does not " swallow his indignation " but in one moment disburses all his credits by disrespect, insolence, or a forced escape. This is one of the reasons why the cyclothyme delinquents show an unpromising prognosis if the number of institutional punishments is taken as a basis. It seems as if the past experiences of the unpleasant consequences of such acts have very little inhibitive influence. The present, aggressive emotions take complete possession of consciousness and derivatively inhibit the already weak perseverative influence of past experiences. Persistent intentions (Einstellungen) according to Kretschmer, Enke, Pfahler, Skawran, and also in our own experience, are very rudimentary in cyclothymes. In terms of Heymans and Wiersma this would mean that cyclothymes of the hypomanic variety are primary and not secondary functioning.[1]

As can be expected, these " labile moods ",[2] " the quick temper ", " naïve, impulsive self-feelings and self-sufficiency ", uninhibited candour when provoked, and lack " of long-thought-out purposefulness, systems and schemes ", frequently make them changeable and fickle in their work as well. The slightest friction with an employer leads to explosive reactions and a change of work. In this way the conditions for a rolling-stone, want of employment and money, and, accordingly, for delinquency, are easily created (vide Cases 1 and 43). With the quicksilver-temperament leading to frequent paltry rows, are combined other tendencies which encourage the frequent change of work; Kretschmer says of them, " Daring, not very carefully chosen undertakings and almost naïve disregard for tact and prudence."[3] They

[1] Re-edited in Heymans' " Ges. Kleinere Schriften ", *Spezielle Psychologie*, pp. 269, 415, etc. Vide also Brugman, *Methoden en Begrippen*, Groningen, 1922 ; T. J. Hugo, *Karakterstudie en Opvoeding*, Pretoria, 1922 ; Wiersma, *Zeitschr. f. Ang. Psychologie*, Bd. 33, p. 146.
[2] The labile moods are emphasized as one of the fundamental qualities of the Integrated or B-type of Jaensch, *Grundzüge*, 147, 264, 323 ; Oeser, *op. cit.*, 191, 195.
[3] *Physique and Character*, p. 131.

resemble an alternating current as compared with a direct current, as Oeser puts it when he compares the B-type with the T-type.[1]

The central quality of these querulous and fiery temperaments is the extreme sthenic self-feelings. These sthenic self-feelings correspond to those of epileptoids in certain respects. The epileptoid, we saw, is incapable of critical self-scrutiny. Even in his egocentric, sugary philosophizing about himself, and in his moralizing, the athletic lacks the real self-knowledge. The sharp antithesis: " I " and " the External World "—" a constant excited self-analysis and comparison " accompanied by self-insufficiency feelings is mainly found in hyperæsthetic leptosomes. Accordingly, the " ego-consciousness ", " a knowledge about the self " as contrasted with " a feeling of the self" characterize the leptosome more than any other type. Cyclothymes have " self-feelings " and not so much an ego-consciousness,[2] " no sharp distinction between ' I ' and the outside world, but a life in the things themselves," " giving themselves up to the mood of the milieu, swinging with it and identifying themselves with it ",[3] with an " almost ludicrous conviction of the value of their own personality ". The hypomanic's self-feelings are "naïve and childlike ". These self-feelings differ essentially from those of the athletics in that they are less coldly calculative towards an aim; less persistent in aggressive intentions; and less pedantically sugary in their verbal manifestations. It is true that many hypomonics in their loud aggressive reaction-waves, may be temporarily blind to the rights and feelings of others.[4] The high spirits, sexual intemperance and superficiality

[1] Oeser, *Zeitschrift f. Psychologie* 112, p. 228.
[2] Many authorities emphasize the *naïvité*, childlike assuming, and unreflectiveness of the hypomanic's self-feelings; Bumke, *Lehrbuch*; pp. 341, 203, etc. We can very well compare the self-feelings or self-consciousness of cyclothymes with those of early childhood, as described by Buhler and Stern, *Das Seelenleben des Jugendlichen*, pp. 44, 100, 146: "The self-consciousness of the child is not a knowing about the self, but a feeling of the self, a willing for himself."
[3] *Physique and Character*, p. 129.
[4] Bumke, *Lehrbuch*, p. 348.

of other hypomanics may, as Wernicke maintains, prejudice their capacity of sympathy and consideration very much. But our experience conforms with the views of Bumke, Kretschmer and others, that the real hypomanic constitution, without epileptoid constitutional admixture, is characterized by naïve, childlike good-nature.[1] Even the aggressive, querulous and choleric persons discussed above, swing back to normal phases of sociable good-nature and humour or comfortable enjoying. We shall be on good biological and psychological grounds, if we constantly compare the hypomanic temperament with the early childhood period with unreflective self-feelings, naïve wilfulness, labile moods, impulsive reactions (" Erstes Trotzalter" of Professor Ch. Bühler),[2] but also with natural good-nature between these reactive waves.

35. *Love of Change and Adventure; " Rough whole-hoggers " ; Undaunted, unreflective giving-themselves-up-to-the-wide world; Lability of Moods and Attitudes; Gangleaders*

This is also a group of cyclothymes nearer to the manic than to the depressive pole of the diathetic range. We can see that this group is intimately related to those discussed in the previous paragraph. The naïve self-feelings and disregard of tact, prudence, and long-thought-out schemes of purposefulness are common to both. But especially the naïve optimism and unreflective, high spirits still to be discussed in succeeding paragraphs, are very important aspects of this group. On the somatic side, we have found as well, that all these hypomanic variants have slight athletic components, such as fair muscularity, well-developed chest, fairly high chin, broad shoulders, fair body-height, etc. This may indicate that the sthenic qualities found in hypomanics and athletics depend on the presence of athletic constitutional elements. The cyclothyme fundaments (such as *naïvité*, sociability) and the schizothyme fundaments (such as perseveration of

---

[1] Bumke, *Lehrbuch*, pp. 203, 348 ; Kretschmer, *Physique and Character*, pp. 135, 244 ; *Deutsche Jur. Zeit.*, 31, p. 785.
[2] *Das Seelenleben des Jugendlichen*, p. 103.

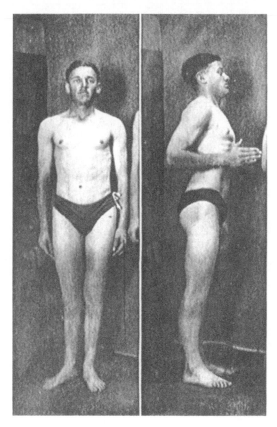

FIG. 43.

[face p. 186

intentions, "social distance"), however, with which the
sthenic attitude is alloyed, lend the sthenic behaviour
a different stamp (Gepräge) in each of these syndromes.
Especially in the present group, athletic components
could always be demonstrated (vide Fig. 43). The following
cases will illustrate our contentions :—

> *Case* 42.—Age 18½ years. When 17 years old convicted
> of theft under false name. One and a half years after that,
> theft of money, fountain pen, etc., from a flat at Durban
> during midnight, flung door in the face of the pursuer,
> tried to go down fire escape, was arrested, and pleaded
> guilty, but asked permission to change from the evening
> dress he wore. Two other convictions of theft of money,
> etc., from flats during same time. Committed to reformatory.
> After eight months escaped in broad daylight by pushing
> a dirt-cart to the dirt-heap and then bolting off. During the
> interview he told me with pleasant enthusiasm that at such
> narrow escapes he " gets a cold feeling on the cheeks, and
> feels electricity in all his limbs ". " Oh, it is simply glorious
> to fly before them." He walked from C.T. to Paarl, where
> he obtained employment on a fish cart ; was hurt, but his
> employer refused to call in medical attendance ; in agony
> of painful arm stole employer's purse and returned to C.T.
> With wounded arm stole close on £100 from flats : " End
> of month and lots of cash flying about," he says. Went
> to Joburg, five counts of theft from flats, some in broad
> daylight when owner of flat in café below, or in bathroom ;
> others at midnight while owner asleep. On one occasion
> owner woke up, "shouted thief and murderer and God knows
> what all." Accused jumped through the window and landed
> on a roof 20 feet below, half-stunned he crept through a
> window into a room, " heard a man snoring and a watch
> ticking," felt about and got a heap of bank-notes with which
> he escaped. Says himself, " A Rolls-Royce life and a Ford
> salary," " the money did fly, by Gosh it did." Very fond of
> cafés and cabarets, with selected girls. When his sexual
> impulse runs high in a romantic situation, he has no scruples
> in satisfying it. Enjoys the adventure of his narrow escapes
> very much. Very boastful to his fellows about his past
> deeds and his sexual excesses. Says : " I have had some
> narrow escapes, some hard times, and some high tides, I have
> slept on the floor of the Ramblers with a newspaper over me,
> and at the Carlton Hotel.[1] I have gone for days without so

---

[1] The Ramblers is a sports pavilion ; the Carlton Hotel is the largest
hotel in Johannesburg.

much as a cup of coffee, my belt tied in to the last link ;
but I have also stolen tons of money in one night." In
many of his flat burglaries he left the door open to show that
somebody had been inside. Always leaves the silver behind,
as he says, for the man to buy food with ; and after a " fat
spoil " gives the Salvation Army a few shillings to ease his
conscience. If he has money, he never sends a beggar away,
" knows what it is to be penniless." In reformatory very
refractory to good order ; in my presence, when asked by
the woodwork officer where another boy was, he answered :
" He went out of the shop because he did not like the smell
of onions." He does not mind punishment, but is annoyed
by all the paraphenalia in connection with it. Says he had
some good intentions formerly, but "for the present, hang
it all ! '' In his letters very self-assertive ; says he did not
drag his name through the mud, but changed it. Tells lies
in boys' court and cheeky when reprimanded. Witty,
boyish, self-feelings. Says all his lies to obtain forbidden
tobacco are entered by God on the Government's account.
At swimming pond, rash overhead diving, more reckless than
energetic.

Somatically : A pyknic with slight athletic signs in
musculature, breadth of shoulders and height of chin.

This case is a fairly typical hypomanic. The following
qualities are outstanding : Undaunted flat expert ; makes
a joke of danger and narrow escapes ; no scruples about
sexual intemperance ; naïve and defiant disregard of
tact, prudence, and long-thought-out schemes of purposefulness and consequences ; social attitude ; a certain
amount of good nature ; extreme self-feelings making
him refractory to disciplinary control, however.[1]

Case 43.—Age 18. With two other boys (vide Case 14)
stole motor-car. The athletic leptosome (Case 14), who had
arranged everything, wanted to look for work. But this
pyknic only wanted to have a good time away from home.
At home he was a bully with his people. In reformatory :
easy-going but with occasional angry reactions when
provoked ; a violent temper ; stands for his rights in boys'
court ; in interview explained that his love of a change and
quick temper had made him change employment five times

[1] Excellent examples—sometimes introspective reports by highly
educated patients—of the real nature of hypomanic self-feelings are
given by J. T. MacCurdy, *The Psychology of Emotion*, London, 1925.

already ; in secret punishment by taller boys for talk about absconding, he jumped in first and received the severest belting.

Somatically : a well-built pyknic.

The love of change in this case brought about loss of work and theft of a car. Lenz [1] gives two examples of pyknic criminals also with a pronounced love of change of occupation. The only occupation at which one of the cases of Lenz remained, was gambling and swindling (Bauernfang), a line wherein change of situations and partners is a daily matter. These are the temperaments Kretschmer speaks of as " wild man of the world, a glutton, a gambler and a debtor ", and yet, "a man, who lived and let live," " unscrupulous," " boisterous passion," " chronic, changeable, fickleness," " unshackled natures," " tendency to superficiality, tactlessness, over-estimation of himself and recklessness," " impulsive, slap-dash, eloquent and changeable as quick-silver." [2]

Case 44.—Age 20 years. With two other boys stole motor-car in front of police station (intentionally), broke into a store-room and took 24 gallons of petrol, 12 containers, and 4 gallons of oil. Wanted to go for a few days' joy-ride for adventure, etc., and then to return the car. But they completely forgot their intention to change the number-plates (compare with Case 14) and were arrested 60 miles from start. Was sent to industrial School when 14 years old, absconded from this school eight times. Addicted to drink occasionally. Had gonorrhœa when committed to reformatory. In reformatory : Sexually very excitable, many tattoos of nude women with sex parts accentuated ; cheerful and hypomanic in his work, good progress, but extremely quickly discouraged when tasks give slight difficulties, then sulks. This lack of persistence, especially in mental tasks, made the impression on me of a sullen temperament at first ;

[1] *Grundriss der Krim. Biol.*, pp. 176, 189 : Enke also found in psycho-technical experiments that pyknics are more impatient and quick to give up a task, in spite of the fact that they start with a world of optimism. The same was found in the sports performances of the B-type by Möckel-mann, *op. cit.*, pp. 36, 40. Vide also, Hoffmann, *Aufbaus*, p. 106.

[2] *Physique and Character*, pp. 132, 160, 243, 221. According to photos, descriptions, etc., the notorious Chicago gang leader, Al Capone, must belong to this group, both somatically and mentally.

but at swimming and sports he showed much energy and enthusiastic cheerfulness; talkative, sociable and cheerful with fellows; on chest tattoo of a ship in full sails indicating his desire to travel; impulsive and unreflective when in company; absconded from reformatory as well, pretended to be ill and, clad in his pyjamas only, escaped over the roof.

In this case the unreflective giving-himself-up-to adventure and to the wide world is the direct cause of his delinquent absconding and motor-thieving. The instability in tedious exertion is also very obvious: difficulties quickly give rise to unpleasant feelings. Enke has demonstrated experimentally that pyknics frequently grow impatient and quickly relinquish a task after some fruitless trials.[1] This is the more striking if one considers the boundless, naïve self-confidence with which they begin. The unpleasant feeling-state which develops when tedious exertion or difficulties defy the pyknic's naïve self-feelings, even retain the hypomanic self-assertiveness, and manifest as a defiant, negative attitude. In some cases, however, a slight undertone of real depressive feelings is reported by Kretschmer in hypomanic temperaments. The lability of emotions and moods, either from enthusiastic, enterprising self-feelings to defiant, angry self-assertion and back again to naïve, pleasant self-feelings; or from naïve exaltation to sudden depression and back again, is a fundamental characteristic of the cyclothyme and of the corresponding type of the Jaensch school: B-type or Integrated type. We have often quoted Kretschmer, and also described typical cases to prove this lability of moods and attitudes. Kretschmer frequently mentions the "labile mood basis", "quick-silver temperament" when he describes the hypomanic, i.e. the more common pyknic variant.[2] Jaensch fully agrees with this in his depictions of the B-type: "Labile and fluctuating moods," "quick-

---

[1] Enke, *Zeit. f. Ang. Psych.*, Bd. 36, pp. 263, 251, 266.
[2] *Physique and Character*, pp. 126, 128. This hypomanic variant of the pyknics, which according to Kretschmer is much more common than the melancholic variant, would therefore correspond to the choleric type of Heymans and Wiersma (*op. cit.*), i.e. the "emotional, primary-functioning, active" combination.

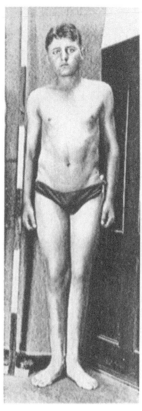

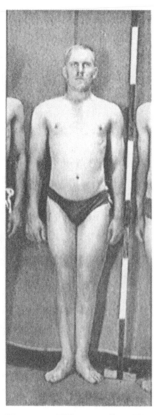

FIG. 44.

FIG. 45. This as well as Fig. 43 gives the gang leader physique type.

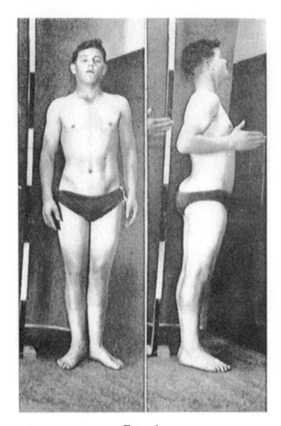

Fig. 46.

[*face p.* 191

silvery," "quick mood changes," "high waves which are quickly smoothed," and do not manifest "the enduring after-effects and summation of stimuli" of the T-basis.[1] The cyclothyme's changeful moods correspond to his lack of persistent (i.e. perseverative) "intentions" or attitudes (Einstellungen). With regard to the mental processes of the hypomanic, Kretschmer says : "Here come out particularly clearly, the lack of system, the way in which he is conditioned by the moment, his childlike abandonment to any impression that is fresh in the mind, to any new idea, the want of judgment, insight, and arrangement, and the consequent lack of construction and absence of guiding ideals : abnormal vigility of interest combined with very little tenacity ".[2] Their overt behaviour as well as their moods, images and ideas change either on the basis of emotional and associative connections or as a result of momentary integrations (harmony, identification) with the environment.[3] There is a "poverty of systematic construction " and of " long-thought-out purposefulness ", on account of this. That is also why they have the naïve, quick, and natural adaptability to new persons and situations, and lack the persistent, revengeful intentions which, in the case of schizoids and epileptoids, may be carried out after a latent period of months.[4]

From these considerations it is obvious that as Kretschmer says, "Mood is all-important, reflection is reduced to a minimum " in the cycloid temperament.

---

[1] W. Jaensch, *Grundzüge*, pp. 145, 264, 165 ; Oeser, *op. cit.*, p. 147.
[2] *Physique and Character*, p. 133.
[3] Möckelmann, *op. cit.*, p. 53. Oeser, pp. 147, 181. It is remarkable how very similar—often identical words—the depictions of the Jaensch and Kretschmer schools are in these fundamental qualities.
[4] The theory of Kretschmer is very interestingly verified by Professor Lange's studies on identical twins (*Verbrechen als Schicksal*, 1929, p. 30), without Professor Lange's knowing it. His Heufelder twins, though very similar, yet show slight differences ; Adolf is more sly, cunning, with roundabout ways creates opportunities, he is cold, mean, secretful. August reflects less, takes an opportunity when it comes, in court explosive and uninhibited, etc. Lange's photographs, etc. indicate that Adolf is more of an athletic (face, profile) while August leans towards pyknic (roundness of face, shallow eyeballs, bald head, dome shape of forehead).

Violent changes of mood or emotions [1] characterize the cycloid, as compared with persistent tensions (motor drivenness) of the epileptoid, and timid excitement of the schizoid. The cyclothyme may, therefore—just as the corresponding B-type of the Jaensch school—be described as " emotional ". This " emotionality " signifies suscepti-bility to simple feelings connected with sensations and images, and to emotions generally, in so far as emotions consist of organic sensations plus accompanying affective tones, and differ from the simple feelings in degree mainly.[2] In physiological terms such a susceptibility to these feeling-states corresponds to what the Jaensch school describes as " vegetatively stigmatized ". Jaensch explains that in this type " the vegetative-autonomic nervous system in all its parts is hyper-excitable ".[3] The excitability of this system (according to Jaensch, Störring, Cannon, etc., intimately connected with emotions) produces the B-type's " integrativeness "—i.e. tendency to momentary complete harmony between the self and environment, and complete harmony between the momentary functions of the self. All functions of the self : sensations, images, intentions, movements, are concordant (in harmony) with the momentary mood or emotion. Sensations, images, intentions, etc., antagonistic to the momentary feeling-state, either change the existent feeling-state or are themselves inhibited from consciousness by the all determining feeling-state. It works, as Rivers

---

[1] Skawran, *Unpublished Lectures*, Pretoria, has worked out a theory according to which emotions and simple feelings are only changes of the existing mood *in statu nascendi*. Emotions are more violent changes of the existing mood, generally as a result of strong fundamental or intentional attitudes being brought into function. Simple feelings are slight changes of the existing mood, usually occasioned by images or sensations simply.

[2] Störring's theory of emotions is that they consist of organic sensa-tions, tensions, excitement, + affective tones which accompany these sensations. He takes simple-feelings accompanying sensations of taste, etc., and images, as also constituted by organic sensations, etc., and their accompanying feeling tones (*Psychologie des Menschlichen Gefühlslebens*, Bonn, 1915 and 1922). Cannon's theory is that emotions and simple feelings derive from processes in the thalamus where the highest autonomic centres are localized (*Bodily Changes*, 1929).

[3] W. Jaensch, *Grundzüge*, pp. 292, 354.

explains, on the "all or none" principle.[1] This gives the queer blindness, one-sidedness, superficiality to the emotional person. And it is on this basis that cyclothymes do things for which they are sorry ; undertake tasks which are super-humanly dangerous or impossible. Their minds work with successive moment complexes ("integration products "),[2] each such complex being a firmly coherent unit by itself, but without strong "intentional" connections between the successive complexes (compare manic flight of ideas). The succession of such moment complexes is relatively strongly determined by the very primitive mechanism of association, feeling-connections, or environmental stimuli, while the schizoid's succession of contents of consciousness is relatively strongly determined by intentions (attitudes, Einstellungen, "perseverative ideas ").[3] That is why the cycloid is much more able than the schizoid, to adapt to, and even to desire a rapid change of situations. We should, as already stated, always compare the temperament of early childhood with that of the cyclothyme. Jaensch has already repeatedly shown that the B-type corresponds to an early childhood phase.

36. " Jolly, light-headed " ; " Naïve optimism " ; Boastful self-sufficiency ; " Enthusiastic talkers " ; Love of jovial company

This cyclothyme variant is, according to Kretschmer, the purest group of hypomanics. They certainly differ constitutionally from the more querulous variant described previously ; but the transitions are so flowing and they have so many constitutionally common radicals that they should in broad divisions all be grouped under hypomanics. As we shall see in a later chapter, the present group may on the neuroglandular side perhaps be more dominated by the thyroid functions, while the other

[1] W. H. R. Rivers, *Instinct and the Unconscious*, Cambridge, 1922.
[2] Oeser, *op. cit.*, and Möckelmann, *op. cit.*
[3] Refer to the investigations of Skawran, Enke, Pfahler, Oeser, Möckelmann, W. Jaensch, etc.

group may have more of the adrenal cortex basis. This would also be supported by the studies of the Jaensch brothers who have indicated the connections between the labile, sociable, naïve, hypomanic B-type, and the Basedow clinical form.[1] The Basedowoid constitution is dominated by thyroid functions. Basedowoid somatic characteristics, such as slight exopthalmos with shining eyes, soft velvety skin, rosy, youthful colour, also seem to be more pronounced in this group of pyknics, than in the querulous and the wild adventurous pyknics. The wild adventurous and reckless variants, however, are nearly on the same biological and psychological basis as the jovial hypomanics. These interrelations and common radicals are clearly demonstrated by the following typical members of the jovial naïve group :—

Case 45.—Age 18. As a leader of two other boys, one a leptosome and the other a pyknic, he stole many motor-cars and left them after their joy-rides through the city's suburbs. Used to fetch girls with these cars, go to lonely places, separate into pairs and practise sexual excesses on a large scale. On other occasions drove with car through the streets making all kinds of mischief. *Inter alia* they tried to knock over the sanitary buckets standing on the edge of the streets at midnight, by just catching them with the car's buffers. When the natives in charge of the buckets placed them away from the edge of the street, the boys loaded the cars with stones to throw at these buckets. One night on returning through a business street, this boy tried to throw the stones still left in the car at a pane of glass. They missed a few, but were full of joy when the stone crashed into one of the large panes. In this way they fractured nine large show-window panes in one night. At the last one they saw a paw-paw through the fractured pane, started a meal and were arrested. In reformatory : Self-opinionated, boisterous, but very generous ; jovial, sociable and good-natured ; very fond of music and singing. In one concert that I attended he took part in nine items ; leader of boys' concerts ; loud in his address, greets me enthusiastically when still at a distance ; boasts pleasantly about his genius for music and recitals ; says he feels sure that he will still do something great for South Africa ; has a fluctuating, but passionate religion ;

[1] W. Jaensch, *Grundzüge*, 1926.

in one of his affectionate letters advocates Christ to one of his old flames and states, " I have changed a lot, damn it, I am entirely another man," also mentions to girl that he is " as fat as a pig " ; he is extremely optimistic in every respect ; naïvely assumes that he is quite handsome and has " much brains " ; argumentative with the purpose of showing the boys what a genius they have the privilege to be with ; when he described the build of his relatives he pantomimed them with a plastic, comical effect.

Somatically : Pyknic but with broad shoulders and fair muscles.

Case 46.—Age 18. Stole motor-car, went for joy-ride till run out of petrol, then took another car. Often changed work, but very fond of sailoring. In interview stated that he very much enjoyed to flee before pursuing police. Does not seek admiration when he drives a car but enjoys the sensation, the speed and the act of controlling the car. Fond of companions, never wants to be alone. Never worried about religion. In reformatory : happy-go-lucky, fond of playing the fool on parade ; full of boyish mischief and naïve optimism ; generous and jovial ; takes his condition with boyish unconcernedness; admits himself in his letters that he is " a hard case ".

Somatically : Dysplastic pyknic (infantile beard, etc.).

Case 47.—Age 19. With a companion stole two horses which he tried to sell. In reformatory : fond of a big meal, smoking and smutty jokes; easy-going, happy-go-lucky ; very sociable and jovial ; quick-tempered but quickly reconciled ; sexually very excitable ; in interview told me that he spent much money on his comrade and also on girls, with some of whom he practised sexual intercourse ; will do anything for money and jovial company ; tears came into his eyes when he stated that he could never have dreamt that matters would turn out as they did. Writes many letters to his home asking for news, photographs, etc., usually in an enthusiastic strain.

Somatically : Pyknic, rather tall with fair muscles.

These cases indicate how the jovial, naïve, optimistic and boyishly playful hypomanic is very liable to certain forms of delinquency. Motor-thieving for the purpose of joy-rides is extremely common with them. It is instructive to compare this type of motor-theft with that of the schizothymes. We saw that the schizothymes steal motor vehicles to keep and use permanently or, in isolated cases, to compensate for their feelings of self-insufficiency by conscious posing and manœuvering before an admiring crowd. The pyknic, we see now, does it for real " joy-riding ". In a naïve way he " identifies " himself with the situation, enjoys the act as such, the sensation, the experience of travelling at a headlong speed. His soul is in the function ; the act becomes spirited (" beseelt ") as Jaensch says of the integrated type.[1] The pyknic does not do it so much because of " long-thought-out purposefulness ", but in a naïve, playful manner. Naïve optimism prevents him from " dreaming that matters would turn out as they did". One of these motor thieves once had a peculiar escape. While he lay under a car endeavouring to disconnect the battery from the keyboard, the owner stepped into the car and drove off, leaving our friend to escape the back wheels and the differential box. The juvenile was very pleased with his interesting escape and did not let this lesson deter him from future risks.

Their self-feelings are of a childish nature. Usually harmless, they may flame into aimless resistance of control. " Purely formal, aimless willing " of early infancy is very near to it. Stern characterizes this type of self-feeling as, "not a knowing of the self, but a feeling of the self, a willing for the self," when analysing the child-mind.[2] In the jovial variety of cyclothymes the self-feelings usually manifest in ludicrously naïve intentions (e.g. to do great things for their country) or ideas (e.g. that they are handsome, and " brainy "). In all this they differ from the epileptoid's "broad complacent moralizing and philosophizing about the self in a sugary manner " by their freshness, naïvité, harmless good nature, and emotional identification with their environment. In their aggressive, fiery reactions they do not show the cold, systematic,

---

[1] Möckelmann, op. cit., indicates that the sport of the B-type is animated (durchseelt) and not a cold, purposeful activity as in many of the T-types. W. Jaensch very strongly emphasizes this intimate emotional integration, and spirit-permeatedness of the B-type's acts and movements (Grundzüge, pp. 141, 162, 271, etc.).

[2] Ch. Bühler, op. cit., pp. 44, 102.

revengefulness, sometimes summating and remaining latent for a long time in epileptoids and schizothymes.[1]

The " live and let live " characteristic, the sociable identification of himself with his co-enjoyers is probably the main cause of delinquency in many pyknics. The last of the three cases given above, is a good example of this. Lenz has already indicated the pyknic's inclination to practise "Bauernfang", i.e. a playful, business-like victimization of green country cabbages by a band of gamblers and swindlers.[2] There is very little long-thought-out, systematic procedure in such a practice. It is essentially a sociable, playful concern where rapid, witty " handling of human beings " and " an eye for the exact moment " are the main necessary qualifications. In our own material, too, pyknics are usually found to prefer escapades in the company of others, with whom the spoils are usually shared, or escapades connected with living beings. They seem to prefer burgling an occupied flat where people are sleeping, to burgling a deserted farmstead or a dark store. In most cases, of course, the pyknic knows how to get sexual, gastronomic, and drink pleasures in return for his money.[3] But his naïve good-nature, sociable relations, and true emotional *rapport* (identification) with his fellow-beings certainly make the pyknic the most generous of the three types.

37. *" Comfortable Enjoyers "*, *Gluttons, Alcoholic Intemperance, Sexual Excesses*

Kretschmer definitely mentions this sub-type, and in many places indicates that comfortable enjoying is an essential characteristic of most cycloids. But the most outspoken form is certainly the hypomanic enjoyer : " a tendency to a certain materialism, to enjoyment,

---

[1] *Physique and Character*, p. 129 ; Jaensch, *op. cit.*, pp. 166, 144, 145, 146.

[2] Lenz, *Grundriss*, pp. 177, 190.

[3] The two cases of criminal pyknics given by Lenz are outstanding in this respect, *op. cit.*, pp. 177, 189. Vide also Kretschmer, *op. cit.*, p. 129.

love, eating and drinking, to a natural seizing of all the good gifts of life ".[1]

> *Case* 48.—Age 17.   Convicted of several counts of fraud. Wrote five letters to stores in the name of his cousin and other people with whom he stayed, asking : (1) 2*s.* polony and 1*s.* biltong ; (2) three tins of jam, two bread, three bags of tobacco, four packets of cigs., two bottles lemonade, 1*s.* sugar, two tins of milk ; (3) two milk, two jam, two bread ; (4) 3*s.* polony ; (5) one jam, one bread, and £1 cash.   In reformatory : extremely easy-going, too lazy even to listen to a story or scrutinize a picture; punishments for tattooing, smuggling tobacco, and theft of food.
> Somatically : Muscular pyknic.

We can also refer to Cases 47, 41 and 42 as examples of this type.   If financial fortune smiles on them, they may in free life become enormously fat.   I have met many of them in South Africa.   Their fatness may create the impression of shortness, but many of them are near to, or even over 6 ft. (183 cm.).   This height—due mainly to strong limbs—and other features such as broad shoulders, high chin, large nose, etc., are clear indications of slight athletic constitutional admixture.[2]   In our delinquent material, too, the real enjoyers always showed slight athletic or athletic-dysplastic constitutional admixture. Lenz[3] speaks of " vegetative ego-assertion " when he deals with the comfortable enjoyer, and the typical example he gives is decidedly a hypomanic pyknic with broad shoulders, fair size of nose and straight, thick hair.   His case must also have a good physique, because he was repeatedly punished for bodily injuries to persons, and had also been employed in such a sturdy line as black-smithing.   The case of Lenz, our own delinquent material, and also cases known to us in private life, prove in another way that these enjoyers must be of a virile and sturdy physique.   All of them are sexually very strongly endowed.

---

[1] *Physique and Character*, pp. 129, 242.

[2] The French leader, Mirabeau, is described by Kretschmer as a glutton, who lived and let live, rocking in comfort.   Kretschmer's plate of him shows a well-built man with particularly strong legs, and a fairly large nose—both indications of athleticism.

[3] Lenz, *Grundriss*, p. 189.

Most of them have had frequent sexual intercourse from their seventeenth year, and I know of a few cases where they indulge in this with their own wives or promiscuously as much as three times per night for a few nights of the week regularly.[1] The slight athletic components in the " comfortable enjoyers " are not at all surprising—in fact, it is in line with our observation that athletics are very prone to be gluttons, especially, of course, the degraded athletic found in reformatories and prisons.   The pyknic, however, is not so much a glutton, but rather a person who " naïvely enjoys " all the good gifts of life.[2]

From the presentations of Lenz, Kretschmer, etc.,[3] it is evident that these " enjoyers " must also fall a ready victim to alcoholic intemperance.   In private life we know of many hypomanic drinkers, and, judged from interviews of our delinquent material, alcoholism seems to be not infrequent in these.   But we are unable to reach definite conclusions in this respect because particulars concerning the pre-reformatory lives of our matcrial have been very unsatisfactorily gleaned and described—mostly by very poorly educated police officers.

As already stated, masculine pyknics of the hypomanic variety are sexually strongly endowed.   Kretschmer lays much emphasis on the general strength of the sexual impulse in pyknic cyclothymes: "The sexual impulses are simple, natural and lively," " in the hypomanic it is generally notably strong," and in the depressive region often over the average.   In cyclothymes we do not find that cleft or disunion between the psychical and somatic aspects of the sex impulse, so frequent in schizothymes. Very few pyknic cyclothymes above 17 years of age are satisfied with masturbation or other pubertial perversions of physical sex, usually practised right up to complete

---

[1] Also Lenz, *op. cit.*, pp. 177, 189.

[2] It is probable that where the noisy hypomanic with very labile moods is dominated by hyperthyroidism and sympathetico-tony, the easy-going, comfortable enjoying cyclothyme has a fair degree of vagotony perhaps intermitted by sympathetico-tony crises (vide Pende, *Konstitution und innere Sekretion*, Leipzig, 1924, p. 23 ; and Cannon, *Bodily Changes*).

[3] Also Bukme, *Lehrbuch*, pp. 650, 349.

manhood by schizothymes. Cases 42, 44, and 45 given above, of hypomanic cyclothymes illustrate this fact. Most of our pyknics who entered the reformatory after 17 years of age, have misbehaved themselves promiscuously.[1] It is difficult to gather enough data for definite conclusions, but judged from evidence and interviews, the pyknics appear to be more discriminative than the athletics in the choice of objects to satisfy their sexual impulses. It is probable that—even if only for a short moment—they also seek their characteristic sociable relations and true emotional *rapport* with their sexual partners. The act must be " spirited " (beseelt) ; it must incorporate the whole emotional personality.[2]

38. *The Depressive Cyclothymes*

In accordance with Kretschmer, we have given the depressive temperamental qualities as : " Quiet, calm, easily depressed, soft-hearted." But they also have the general qualities of cyclothymes, viz. " Sociable, good-natured, friendly, genial". It is already apparent from these combinations that this variant of the cyclothymes will not be inclined towards delinquency of a serious nature. Kretschmer speaks of them in these positive terms : " They can raise themselves from the bottom rung, through their assiduity, conscientiousness, and dependableness, their quiet practical outlook, goodness of heart, affable friendliness, and personal fidelity, to the position of a kind of revered, indispensable, true old factotum, beloved of all." He also mentions " energetic perseverance ", " cautious, all-too-soft natures, tendency to take things too much to heart ", " playing an honourable rôle in more protected situations."

[1] The two cases of Lenz show a remarkable, promiscuously satisfied sexual impulse, *op. cit.*, pp. 177, 189.

[2] Jaensch, *Grundzüge*, pp. 292, 354, 357 ; Möckelmann, *op. cit.* It is noteworthy that the short legs of pyknics are probably due to an early involution of the pineal and other infantile glands, which go parallel with the too early rise of the gonads. Cf. Pende (p. 51),

Cases of an unmixed depressed temperament are very rare in our material. The few cases who tended in this direction, showed many qualities in common with the hypomanic variants, such as naïve, jovial, sociable, good nature in company. But they differ fundamentally from the hypomanics in their lack of sthenic self-feelings. In their delinquent behaviour, and their attitude towards the court and their fellows in free life, and also in the reformatory, they miss all overbearance, loud initiative and self-sufficient leadership. In this respect they remind one very strongly of leptosomes. But they differ from leptosomes in a much freer, more sociable and emotionally true mixing with their momentary environment [1] :—

Case 49.—Age 19. Convicted of several thefts from flats. In most cases these flats were occupied by women. When charged, he confessed all his burglaries, including those unknown to the authorities. Asks the court's pardon, states that he had to do something for food, could not find work. In reformatory : Submissive, fond of all sorts of music ; laughs readily and heartily when his company encourages it ; weak self-assertion in boys' court. Careful and neat at psychotechnical tasks ; unreflective in company.

Somatically : Pyknic, but lean, fairly small eyes and thin muscles.

The delinquent acts of this group are usually more exogenously than endogenously determined : force of circumstances, influence of stronger personalities, etc. In connection herewith there is a peculiar type of murder sometimes committed by more depressed cyclothymes. Böhmer [2] gives an instance where such a pyknic suddenly shot his two children and seriously injured himself after he had reflected for a short while about his unhappy home conditions. His first idea was suicide, and only after that

who found hyper-sexual criminals to be generally of the brevilineus physique. M. J. Breitmann (*Archives de criminologie et de médecine légale*, Kharkoff, 1927, p. 1250) comes to the same conclusion. Vide also Berman, *op, cit.*, p. 99.
[1] Bumke gives an outstanding instance of such a person who sobbingly sought for sociable company ; there he conversed with spirited pleasure, only to go home again and continue his crying, *Lehrbuch*, p. 205.
[2] *Monatschrift* 1928, p. 208.

it occurred to him that he could take his beloved children with him into death. This kind of love-murder we have also described in leptosomes, where, however, the sentimental idealistic aspect is more prominent than in these pyknics who are dominated by the momentary depressed mood.

39. *Connections between Repressive Pole of Cyclothymes and the Leptosomic Constitution*

(a) *Temperament.*

As stated, we have not had many depressed pyknics in our delinquent material. But we have especially endeavoured to observe members of this group in private life. Our observations in both fields have led us to the tentative conclusion that there are intimate biophysiological and psychological connections and flowing transitions between the depressed pyknic and the asthenic schizothyme. This fits in very well with, and completes our " Triangle of Temperaments " (para. 58). We have already seen some similarities between these two groups in the asthenic attitude towards the human environment and in the love-murders. The asthenic attitude, common to both groups, is of utmost theoretical importance, as we shall see when we deal with the biophysiological similarities. Kretschmer has already shown that : " The hypomanic tends towards the sthenic life-attitude, towards pleasure and anger, naïve, imperturbable self-feelings and optimism, an almost ludicrous conviction of own value and own ability ; the melancholic cyclothyme on the contrary, towards a sense of failure, modesty, lack of self-confidence and enterprising courage, self-abasement, sense of guilt, and long depressive reactions." [1] He also shows that the tender hyperæsthetics cannot stand the medium coarseness of life, are easily wounded psychically, tend strongly towards asthenic experiencing, the most harsh

[1] *Med. Psychologie*, p. 194 ; E. Wexberg, " Zur Klinik und Pathogenese der leichten Depressionszustände," *Zeits. f. Neur. und Psych.*, Bd. 112, 1928, p. 565.

insufficiency-feelings, autistic flight from reality, etc. Moreover, a narrowing to an egocentric limit of the capacity to feel with others, with a grotesque measure of presumption, and self-adulation, as well as contempt and ignoring of the environment, inconsiderate and hypertensioned sthenic experiencing and action, is the opposite of the hyperæsthete's asthenic attitude.[1] Kretschmer has, however, not connected this asthenic-sthenic polarity with a somatic basis. But it is obvious that with slight modifications this sthenic opposite of the asthenic hyperæsthete corresponds to the epileptoid temperament which is mainly connected with the athletic habitus. In descriptions of the depressed pole of cyclothymes in his main works,[2] Kretschmer frequently uses characterizations which are almost equally applicable to the leptosome as described by us : " Cat that walks by itself," " slight tendency to hypochondriacal eccentricity," " did not pay much attention to girls, he was afraid they would want to marry him," " belongs to no societies," " faithful circle of friends," " books have been his best friends," " could not bear a rapid change to new situations," " live their lives quietly and in contemplation," " commenced brooding," " a little embarrassed and difficult when he is in a large gathering of people or if a stranger comes across his path," " a certain anxiousness and shyness is found with many cycloid-depressive natures," " energetic perseverance and conscientiousness."

Kretschmer also characterizes certain schizoid forms as " constitutionally depressed ", differing from the real depressives in so far only as they are more distrustful and nervous.[3] W. Jaensch[4] repeatedly mentions that " depressions, anxiety-states and obsessions " are common experiences of tetany patients, and that these moods are

[1] *Med. Psych.*, p. 195.
[2] *Physique and Character*, pp. 126, 141, 142, 143, 134, 168. Vide also his statement about the connections between the schizothyme hyperæsthetic and the cyclothymic, soft, melancholic in sensitive paranoia on which he is a recognized authority (*Med. Psychologie*, pp. 199, 62).
[3] *Physique and Character*, 1925, p. 168.
[4] *Grundzüge*, pp. 126, 427, 460, etc.

favoured by the one-sided presence of the T-basis. Jaensch himself acknowledges—and we too shall indicate this still more fully in the following chapter—that the T-basis in its purest form (calcium shortage in nerve-chemistry, and hypo-function of the parathyroid gland) corresponds to Kretschmer's typical schizo-biotype. Wexberg's [1] analysis of slight depression-states, also throws much light on this problem. He subdivides these depressions into cycloid-, schizoid-, constitutional- (i.e. chronic), climacteric-, cerebral disease- and psychogenic-depressions. With the exception of the cycloid and climacteric varieties, Wexberg maintains that schizoid traits predominate in all these depressions. Anxiety and insufficiency-feelings form the nucleus of all depressions. The depressions with a schizoid basis differ from those with a cycloid basis, mainly in the tendency of the former to hypochondriacal and paranoid traits. Such schizo-qualities as " habitual anxiousness, shyness, reserve, excitability " have in many depressions already from the beginning characterized the pre-morbid lives of the patients. Sexually-coloured anxieties and insufficiency-feelings are also very frequent. Wexberg accordingly concludes: " Owing to this multiplicity of constitutional bases ' Depression-states ' completely lose the nature of a nosological unity, and become a signification for a psycho-pathological symptom complex without a unitary etiology, and for a reaction-type which can develop in diverse frameworks." The flowing transitions between constitutional depression and sensitive paranoia are also recognized by Bumke. The same author believes that certain periodic depressions in schizophrenic patients can sometimes make the differential diagnosis between schizophrenia and manic-depression almost impossible. [2]

(b) *Physique.*

On the somatic and physiological side there are many indications, too, of a close relationship between the

---

[1] Wexberg, *Zt. f. Neur. und Psych.*, Bd. 112, p. 547.
[2] Bumke, *Lehrbuch*, pp. 371 and 729.

depressive pole of cyclothymes and the asthenic schizo-thymes. In the few cases of delinquent cyclothymes who are inclined towards the depressive pole, we have almost always observed some indications of leptosomic con-stitutional admixture : deep-seated, small eyes without the lustre and vigour of the protruding eyes (*protrusio bulborum*) so frequently met with in hypomanics ; pointed chin (perhaps somewhat receding) without strong bony and fatty lateral projection of the lower jaw, and thus bringing the front-view circumference of the face nearer to the shortened egg-shape ; nose thin rather than snubbed and with tip drawn downwards ; more delicate bones, joints, and muscles ; shoulders narrower; relatively small skull circumference, etc. The same observations were made on a few individuals known to us in private life. Though the number of cases is not enough to conclude from it dogmatically, we have found cases where such " soft " pyknics have blood relatives with a pronounced leptosomic physique—an indication of the hereditary " impurity " of the constitution of such depressive pyknics. Without suggesting any hypothesis, Kretschmer [1] himself has given instances indicating empirical connections between the leptosome (asthenic) physique and the depressive psychical constitution. In his chapter on the building of the constitution he gives the following example of a mixed constitution : " A typical obstructed depression " with an " almost pure asthenic " physique. In the same chapter he gives another case of " a decided asthenic appearance ", " narrow chest and a curvature of the spine (kyphosis) ", " in combination with a simple inhibited depression ". In accordance with his demonstration of schizoid elements in many depressions, Wexberg [2] also found leptosomic somatical factors in these depressions. Leptosomes predominated in the schizoid-, constitutional (i.e. chronic) and in the psychogenic depressions. Athletics were seldom in all forms. But pyknics predominated in cycloid- and climacteric-

---

[1] *Physique and Character*, pp. 96, 104.
[2] Wexberg, *op. cit.*

depressions, and were also present in the other forms to such a degree that these forms cannot be interpreted as pure schizoidy. Wexberg also mentions that Professor J. Lange found one pyknic and nine asthenics among eleven psychogenic depressions.

Zeckel [1] of the Groningen clinic, on the basis of his own research and a review of all the more important German, English, and American researches, concludes that a lowering of the basal metabolism is common to depression and schizophrenia. In a similar manner Teenstra [2] of the same clinic comes to the conclusion that a hyperglycæmia is common to depression and schizophrenia. Both these conclusions indicate important, mutual physiological conditions in these two clinical forms. But particularly the conclusion of Teenstra with regard to glycæmia, which, in the light of Cannon's researches, may be due to a hyper-function of the adrenal medulla (adrenalin), and accordingly to chronic fear,[3] fits in admirably with our contention that in asthenics the nerve excitement discharges into autonomic fear centres. It is probable that the fear-conditions (or in a characterological form : " feeling of insecurity ", " asthenic experiencing ") form the nucleus of both forms. But this nucleus is manifested differently when involved in the different constitutions : it is autistic, eccentric, perseverative, in the leptosomic constitution; and sociable, naïve, emotional, in the pyknic constitution. Somatically the absence of athletic elements, especially the musculature, is striking in both forms. This may— as we explained in connection with the difference between athletics and leptosomes in the schizothymes—produce

---

[1] *Grondstofwisseling by Psychosen*, Groningen, 1929.

[2] *Bloedsuikergehalt by Melancholie en Schizophrenie*, Groningen, 1929.

[3] Cannon (*Bodily Changes*, 1929) found adrenalin secretions as an accompaniment of various emotions, i.e. fear and anger. Other researches seem to indicate that adrenalin alone without the adrenal cortex secretion is present in fear, while in anger the cortex secretion plays a determining rôle (Berman, Pende, Teenstra, etc.). It is, as Jaensch mentions, doubtful whether the endocrine organs, in this parallelism, are not themselves of secondary importance. It may be that the autonomic centres in the thalamus-striatum innervate the endocrine organs regulatively.

the absence of aggressive tensions (muscular tonus) in the extreme depressive. In the cyclothyme group, therefore, as well as in the schizothyme group, the sthenic form of experiencing seems to go with musculature, broad shoulders and other athletic constitutional factors, while asthenic experiencing seems to go with lack of musculature, fine bones and other asthenic physique factors. In terms of endocrine functions, the asthenic-sthenic proportions probably correlate with hypo- and hyper-activity of the adrenal cortex and the anterior-pituitary (in men at least).[1]

SUMMARY OF CONCLUSIONS

1. The hypomanic variants of the cyclo-type are constitutionally related to athletics, as indicated in my triangle.

2. Querulants and self-feeling cholerics with occasional serious aggressions are frequent in our hypomanic delinquents. It is possible that their constitutions are not quite pure.

3. The undaunted adventurers, gang-leaders and changeful, rough whole-hoggers figure largely in youthful delinquents. Athletic constitutional factors are always found in them.

4. Jovial optimists and sociable enjoyers are flowingly connected with the foregoing groups. They usually have athletic physical qualities as well, but may perhaps be more dominated by the thyroid, while the former may be more adrenal cortex centred.

5. In all these variants the delinquency usually is the direct outcome of their temperaments : momentary aggressions, sensational joy-rides with stolen motors, criminal gangs, money wasters, sexual excesses, enjoyers, alcoholic intemperance.

6. In these temperaments, as well as in the schizo-type, outlined in previous chapters there are close correspondences with the types of Jaensch.

7. Depressive variants are not frequent in delinquents. Moreover, their delinquency is mainly exogenously determined.

8. The depressive variants manifest asthenic qualities in temperament as well as in physique. This is explained by, and further completes our triangle.

[1] Berman, Pende.

CHAPTER VII

MENTAL (INCLUDING DELINQUENT) QUALITIES OF SOME DYSPLASTIC TYPES

40. *Dysplastic Factors in the Three Main Types*

In para. 13 we contended that dysplasias (physical manifestations of dysglandularisms) should prove very significant in all abnormal personalities of whom criminals, psychopaths, etc., are certainly sub-groups. Unfortunately, the dysplastic group is very heterogeneous, and dysplastic types have not been worked out definitely enough or in sufficient detail. We can, therefore, give only very vague co-ordinations between dysplasias and crime, or dysplastic types and delinquent types.

In our material we frequently found dysplasias, though only in very few cases were these dysplastic, somatic qualities so pronounced that they blurred or overruled the qualities according to which the cases can be classified into the three main constitutional types. But even where the cases can still be classified, and the dysplastic qualities merely serve as an additional stigmatization, these qualities are of major importance as the following indicates :—

(a) *Dysplastic Leptosomes.*

The extreme asthenic physique is nothing but a dysplasia or a dysglandularism.

It is connected with dysfunctions of the thymus (hyper) and the parathyroid (hypo) endocrine organs. The delinquencies, such as parasitism, slyness, etc., connected with such extreme atonicity must, therefore, be mainly brought into relation with the dysplastic conditions. The homosexuality of this type and of the eunuchoid variants of the leptosomic type are definitely related to dys-glandularisms. In fact, Kronfeld, Lenz, and we ourselves

(Cases 6, 12, 50) have found many connections between homosexuality, infantile sex-manifestations, etc., on the one hand, and dysplastic conditions on the other hand.

(b) *Dysplastic Athletics.*

Kreyenberg has shown that in epileptic and in epileptoid athletics dysplastic conditions are remarkably frequent. We have indicated in our chapter on athletics that epileptoid hypertensions probably depend, either on constitutional extremes (hyperpituitary), or on mixtures and dysglandularisms. In the Düsseldorf mass-murderer, and in other prominent athletic criminals, sexual abnormalities—probably with somatic correlates—are of central importance. In this way the dysplastic (dysglandular) conditions, though not predominant in the physique, are still intimately connected with the delinquency. The athletic dysplastics, i.e. in whom not the athletic but the dysplastic (plump, ill-proportioned, ugly, and pasty) physique elements dominate already, we shall discuss in the dysplastic group below.

(c) *Dysplastic Pyknics.*

According to Kretschmer pyknics are not much inclined towards dysglandularisms. Nevertheless, we believe to have found some dysplastic features in certain cyclo-temperaments: the comparatively coarse head-hair, long legs, and pronounced eyebrows in some professional quarrellers; infantile, hypoplastic physical qualities in some of the melancholic variants; and also dysglandular adiposity in certain cases of extreme vagotonic enjoyers (vegetators, vide Fig. 26), all seem to indicate dysplastic conditions also in pyknics.

41. *Feminisms*

In many leptosomes of eunuchoid-like build (Case Nos. 6, 50) feminine temperament-qualities are displayed, such as lack of manly self-assertion, susceptibility to sexual abuse by other boys, and to influence generally, small vanities, etc. In our material we had no pronounced cases of feminism. Lenz and Kronfeld give excellent examples of such inter-sexuality, showing both in the physique and in the mind. The following is a case found in our own material, which illustrates some of the main principles (vide also Cases 6, 54).

Case 50.—Age 17½ years. Had to deliver a message at a house; found owner not at home, entered and stole wristlet watch which he wore when arrested. On previous occasion stole another watch, also on the impulse of the moment, when alone in his uncle's house. Under the influence of taller and older boy stole various articles, such as ties, safety-razors, etc. Very fond of company and bioscopes. For this purpose frequently stole money from parents and acquaintances.

Usually very sorry after deed committed, sometimes even returning articles stolen under tempting circumstances. Frequent change of work; preferred motor-mechanics, because fond of fine cars.

In reformatory: inclined to be vain and to display; fond of finding out secrets; prefers gentle games, played in neat attire; easily put to shame and blushes very quickly; easily brought to tears; sociable and obedient; good intentions, but lacks tenacity; unreliable. My finding: Sensitive sense of honour; blushes remarkably, e.g. when previous career referred to, or when asked to be photographed nakedly. In tests tried hard to make a good impression, but not much tenacity. Neat and fond of good clothes. Very shy towards girls, never any love-relations with them. Letters: A very girlish, regular, school-handwriting; goody-goody ideas; sorry about his past, and has many good intentions; superficially religious; intimate with his mother.

Physique: Ruddy cheeks; soft, velvety skin; soft, sentimental eyes; round, soft facial lines. Hair-line on forehead characteristically feminine curve from ear to ear, without corners on sides of forehead.[1] No beard so far. Narrow shoulders, if compared with broad hips; generously curved contour of hips; very long legs if compared with length of trunk (vide Fig. 27); characteristically feminine localization of genital hair.

Owing to insufficient material we cannot elaborate on any pronounced dysplastic conditions of which feminism

[1] Lenz, *Grundriss*, p. 116.

is one ; but we have to point out, nevertheless, that the feminine factors are of great help in explaining such cases as the foregoing one. The boy, though near the leptosomic physique type (hip-shoulder proportion, length of legs, weak secondary hair), and leptosomic temperament (ego-conscious sensitivity, susceptibility to influences) shows many mental and physical qualities which are not quite reconcilable with the leptosomic type : on the physique side, his ruddy cheeks, susceptibility to blushing, his round, soft facial and body lines, and absence of lean, bony body ; on the mental side, extreme love of company, lack of persistence, etc. If the feminine constitutional factors, however, are taken into consideration as well, the physique, temperament, and delinquent behaviour at once become much plainer. Thus not only in extreme cases of homosexuality, or sexual perversions are feministic constitutional factors very significant, but also in less pronounced feminisms in physique, temperament, and delinquency.

42. *Infantilism and hypoplasias*

Cases of infantilism are frequently found in the following form : backwardness of physiological, temperamental, and sometimes intelligence age, if compared with the chronological (vide Figs. 20, 21). But we do not want to deal with these exhaustively either, because they have been fully treated by Healy, Burt,[1] and others. We need only state that these infantiles show the following mental and delinquent qualities :—Susceptibility to the influence of more robust fellows ; weak physical powers as required in the labour-market and as tested by the ergograph (vide Fig. 29*d*, *e*) ; a pronounced form of unpremeditative, naïve, aimlessness (puerilism) [2] ; weak tenacity ; change-fulness. As such the infantile qualities only complicate

---

[1] Burt, *The Young Delinquent*, p. 210 ; Healy, *The Individual Delinquent*, p. 237.
[2] Compare Kretschmer, *Über Hysterie*, 1927, pp. 23, 39. Hysterical qualities connected with infantilisms and feminisms are very frequent in our material.

the typological characteristics of these cases, because, in spite of the infantilisms and temperament, many of them can still be classified into the three main types of physique and temperament.

As far as hypoplasias are concerned, we found an all-round hypoplasia in a few cases. Skawran has observed more or less the same in adults, and has termed them " doll-type ". At present he is engaged on a more intensive investigation of these adult cases, and believes that they may show a particular mental type. Our juvenile cases are so built that they give the impression of miniature editions of the normal adult type (vide Figs. 16, 17, 18). Although the number of such cases in our material is too small to reach definite conclusions, it seems as if the all-round hypoplastic types, just as in the case of many of the infantilistic types, can still be classified into the three main physique and temperament types, complicated, naturally, by the corresponding physique and temperament infantilisms. This tentative conclusion must be illustrated by the following three cases : a miniature leptosome, a a miniature athletic, and a miniature pyknic, respectively :—

Case 51.—Age 16 years. Father and mother divorced. Boy retained by father, but absconded to his mother several times ; even when committed to industrial school, he persuaded other boys to accompany him, and absconded. Extremely attached to his mother, the best treatment by his stepmother or by industrial school cannot keep him from absconding. Stole money and food for this purpose. In reformatory : Very sad that he cannot go to his mother and stay with her. Easily influenced and abused by bigger boys. Victim of persistent smoking. My findings : A tiny, lean, and miniature leptosome (height 148 cm., weight 40 Kg., vide Fig. 16) ; too weak to pull ergograph even with 4 Kg. (usual weight 5 Kg.) ; easily moved to tears ; very timid, reserved, and submissive. Told me that he had absconded from industrial school because boys maltreated him. (In revenge would like to put prickly pear thorns in their beds ! But would not prefer to punish them more drastically.) Unreflective, but not impulsive ; rather fatalistic. On football field a weakling—neither pluck nor power. He has neither beard nor secondary hair. Nipples totally infantile.

Case 52.—Age 19 years. Stole revolver and tools from the store where he worked. Went to police and asked them to lock him up, because he had stolen something. Father states that the boy is wayward, and anxious to distinguish himself as his brothers did (three of them had been in reformatories), wants to get away from his home town by teasing the police. On previous occasions had already shown disrespect to police officers. Only occupation is swimming, dived into water so often and from such a height that his ear-drums were affected. My finding : absolutely aimless ; never worries about future or serious life-ideals ; superficial in tests, conversation, and behaviour. Always ready to join in with whatever is proposed by his fellows ; silly boyishness (puerilism). Immense energy at games and play, at swimming pond indefatigable diving, swimming, and running without forethought or care. Frequent punishment for carelessness, mischief and disrespect. In letters also boyish boldness, but silly ideas ; says " Things are pretty slack at the reformatory now, because inmates have decreased from 112 to 100 " ; boasts to his sister that he courted a girl for nine years, and therefore knows what is what. Tells me that he stole many cars for joy-rides, together with other boys, slipped into bioscopes without tickets, and stole sweets from stores, etc. Somatically a miniature athletic (height 158 cm.), well-proportioned, with exceptionally fine well-toned muscles, but no beard whatsoever, and weak secondary hair (vide Fig. 17).

Case 53.—Age 16 years. Committed to reformatory for repeated absconding from industrial school. Committed to industrial school because beyond parents' control. Played truant from school for days. Stole watch from a girl. In reformatory : totally intractable ; the following major offences recorded in $2\frac{1}{2}$ years (minor lapses without number) : persistent neglect of kit ; smoking innumerable times ; spitefully breaking a pane ; dishonesty ; filthy language ; persistent insubordination, losing boots several times ; misconduct during divine service ; in possession of money ; disrespect and gross insolence several times ; cruelty to a cat ; theft of money ; theft of food ; out of dormitory at night. My finding : a miniature pyknic, no secondary hair (height 151 cm., weight 41 Kg. ; vide Fig. 18). Very boyishly mischievous ; sociable ; happy-go-lucky ; jovial ; unreflective ; says and does things before he thinks ; well pleased with life at the reformatory—frankly states that he has tobacco hidden in his bed. Boyishly enthusiastic about my colleague's motor-cycle, at once mounted it (without permission) where it stood, took handles and said beamingly " Durban–Johburg handicap ".

We accordingly submit the tentative conclusion that such " miniature editions " (proportionate hypoplasia) of the three main types, apart from real infantile mental characteristics, also seem to show some mental resemblances to the typical characteristics of the main types to which they correspond.

43. *Athletic Dysplastics*

(a) *Plump, pasty.*

Under these we understand a heterogeneous group of ill-proportioned, plump, coarse-skinned, thick hair-fibred, massive physiques, all of whom, however, have athletic factors in their constitutions as well. Some, or all of the following athletic constitutional qualities are observed in them: coarse-fibred head-hair; fair skeletal musculature; broad shoulders; heavy bones and joints; long legs, relative to length of trunk; deep-seated, small eyes (tetanoid) etc. The one group (Figs. 22, 23) seems to be—as we indicated in para. 13 (*e*)—nearer the usual athletic physique, only more plump and ill-proportioned. Some of these also seem to have infantile and feminine somatic qualities (Figs. 20, 21 (centre), and 22). The second group are shorter and muscularly thick-set, so that they may sometimes be confused with athletic-pyknic mixtures (Figs 24, 25 ; vide also Case 59(*a*)).

In our material both these groups, particularly the first group, unmistakably manifested the epileptic-temperament of Kretschmer and Mauz, as opposed to the epileptoid hypertensions : they are mostly fairly inactive, sluggish, godwilled dependent, fatalistic, syrupy (süsslich) adhesive, ego-centric, etc.[1] When infantile or feminoid constitutional factors are also present, the fundamental characteristics remain more or less the same, but are complicated by

[1] *Med. Psych.*, p. 222.

such alloys. The following cases, taken from this first group, must prove and illustrate our contention :—

Case 54.—Age 19 years. Took wallet with £12 from a room, when the occupant, to whom he had been sent with a message, left him alone in the room for a few minutes. When arrested, apologized, stating that bad companions had misled him. Wanted to repay money in instalments ; had bought clothes with it. Previous conviction for theft of bicycle. Does not give trouble to parents, but often changed work ; inclined to be lazy. In reformatory : apathetic, submissive and easily led. Addicted to self-abuse, and fond of listening to smutty jokes, negligent, unreliable. My findings : apathetic, and sluggish ; colourless ; little initiative ; easily persuaded ; the opposite of a strong character ; passive egotism. In interview : frequent, undetected store-breaking, under the leadership of other boys ; always took whatever useful articles he found. Had never had any relations with girls, and showed no interest in sport. Physique : fairly tall, ill-proportioned athletic ; distinct feminoid constitutional qualities, e.g. very weak secondary hair on face, hip-shoulder proportions, etc. (vide Fig. 22).

Case 55.—Age 17½ years. With two other boys stole large quantities of clothing material from a factory where they were employed. Other two boys conducted their case in such a way that they were acquitted, and this boy, on account of confessions, given all the blame. Stole, over a period of two months, by frequently wrapping material round his body, underneath his clothes. Parents find him to be obedient and home-loving, but easily persuaded. In court dull-witted. In reformatory : normal intelligence, but of a dreamy disposition ; no interest in sport ; sometimes found in tears with no obvious reason; very weak resistance to temptation (petty stealing and persuasion by others). My finding : strange, sugary smile when speaking ; fairly sluggish and dependent ; wandering, shallow attention ; no interest in girls, but fond of dogs, homely hobbies, and his younger brothers and sisters. Physique : fairly tall athletic, but somewhat ill-proportioned, plump ; curved upper-spine (vide Fig. 23).

Case 56.—Age 16½ years. Committed to industrial school for stealing bicycle and for truancy. From industrial school absconded five times in six months, or nine times in nine months. Principal of school reports that boy is very honest and upright, but unable to resist the impulse. Boy himself very unhappy and fatalistic about it, wants to be locked up to get peace of mind. My finding: Friendly, good-natured, somewhat shy smile; cumbersome; un-concerned; does not smoke, because too difficult to obtain tobacco; teased by other boys. Physique: athletic dysplastic, with infantile stigmata, e.g. shape of head (vide Figs. 20, 21 centre).

These cases certainly have much in common with the epileptic syndrome. They have the typical epileptic mental qualities, and seem to be fairly free from epileptoid crises. Even when they act "drivenly", as in the absconding of Case 56, they rarely come to aggressive violence, and they very much accentuate their helpless-ness, in resisting these weaknesses ("dagegen anzu-kämpfen"). Our results agree with those of Kreyenberg, who found that in actual epileptic materal, the dysplastics are more inclined to the "epileptic" character, as described by Kretschmer; and the athletics more to the "epileptoid" character.[1] In Delbrück's terms the epileptics tend more towards the "boundness" pole, while the epileptoids (athletics) more towards the "drivenness" pole.[2]

The second group of athletic-dysplastics, who are somewhat shorter and muscularly thick-set, can, as we have mentioned, sometimes be easily confused with athletic pyknics. Very important criteria for differentiating are the following: the height, though below that of the average athletic, always seems to be from 1–3 cm. above that of the pyknic averages; length of legs, 1–3½ cm. above pyknic averages; skin matt, pasty, and coarse; hair coarse-fibred and low hair-line on forehead. It is necessary, however, to indicate here that there seem to be gradual transitions, both somatically and mentally from this group to some forms of hypomanic querulants, and passive vegetatives, as found in the pyknic group (vide Figs. 44, 26, 42).

My material is too heterogenous and small in this respect to reach definite generalizations. This group nevertheless appears to have many of the fundamental

[1] Kreyenberg, *op. cit.*; Kretschmer, *Med. Psych.*, p. 222.
[2] Delbrück, *op. cit.*

epileptic (not epileptoid) temperament-qualities of Kretschmer, Kreyenberg, and others, e.g. fatalism towards their delinquent inclinations, matter-of-fact outlook, susceptibility to influences, uncritical religiousness. Occasionally they also react angrily, but, as far as we could observe, it is more in the nature of reactive anger, than an endogenous crisis of irritability. A striking quality observed by us, and which should be further investigated, is the following : the relative frequency (three out of eight) of incest in this group. The following examples will illustrate the tentative statements made above :—

Case 57.—Age 17 years. Under the leadership of another boy (Case 61) stole motor-cycle, rode on pillion. Frequent store-breaking and absconding from industrial school. Always stole under leadership of others, and usually food, tobacco, money in order to go to bioscopes. Absconding for fear of punishment (for sums, previous absconding, and negligence). In reformatory : sluggish ; unconcerned ; fond of a big meal ; friendly ; susceptible to influences ; extremely easy-going ; very matter-of-fact ; when he took off his boots, he said resignedly : " The thick government stockings make one's feet smelly." Takes his own delinquency fatalistically, does not consider it as something serious ; only sorry that he was always so easily found out. Athletic dysplastic (vide Fig. 25) ; height 167·5 cm., pasty skin, coarse-fibred head-hair, reaching low down on forehead, weak beard and other secondary hair ; bridge of nose broad and low ; broad shoulders ; relatively long legs.

Case 58.—Age 18 years. Very calmly and deliberately persuaded his sister, 16 years old, to allow him sexual intercourse with her, which he repeated five times in one month. Girl became pregnant. Another sister, older than boy, is epileptic. My observations : Boy very matter-of-fact. Writes home to describe his journey in a calm manner, as if nothing extraordinary had happened. In interview stated that somebody else was guilty for his sister's pregnancy, but that he took the blame to protect her. Feels quite pleased with himself and with his state in the reformatory. Physique : athletic dysplastic (vide Fig. 24) ; coarse hair, growing low down over the forehead ; matt, pasty skin ; medium height, 167 cm.

Case 59.—Age 19 years. Very calmly and deliberately enticed his sister 15 years old, to sexual intercourse with

him.   Repeated this six times in the course of ten days.
Girl became pregnant.   When accused after birth of child,
he acknowledged his guilt and asked for forgiveness.   In
reformatory extremely fond of eating ; sometimes bad-
tempered.   Keen on boxing ; very easy-going.   Our finding :
Occasional manifestations of anger, e.g. when tests too
difficult, or when another boy jumps upon him in swimming
pond by accident.   Dull, easy-going, but friendly and good-
natured towards us.   In his letters to his home very pathetic
and intimate.   Good intentions, will take up boxing to earn
his mother a living, does not mind if his face is bruised
for mother.   Thankfully penitent and religious, often
sentimental.   In interview stated that he is very much
ashamed of himself, and that, with God's help, he would
lead a better life henceforth.   Physique : extremely muscular,
but fairly short and plump (height 172 cm.).   Secondary
hair weakly developed ; matt skin ; small, dull eyes ;
relatively long legs.

All these plump, pasty athletics are inclined to be
sluggish, syrupy, god-willed, dependent, etc.   In daily
life, too, we have frequently met them.   Then, apart
from the sluggish, dependent attitude, they are usually
hyper-religious and may be students with calm application.
Sexual abnormalities, such as incest, sodomy (with
animals) relations with natives and coloured people,
seem to be generally frequent in these groups.   In our
delinquent material of plump, pasty athletics, we have
also very frequently found dagga-smokers.   This drug-
stimulant temporarily raises them from their " bound "
sluggishness to a state of self-confident excitement (some
what similar to the effects of opium).

(b) Plump Musculars.

The last case, described above, manifests occasional
angry reactions.   This seems to go with the extremely
muscular, though plump, thick-set physique.   Kreyenberg,[1]
makes a difference between the plump, pasty athletics,
and the plump muscular athletics.   We have treated
the plump, pasty athletics, particularly in cases of
marked plumpness and pastiness, under these athletic

[1] Kreyenberg, op. cit.

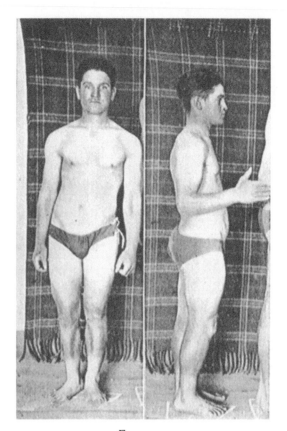

FIG. 47.

[*face p.* 218

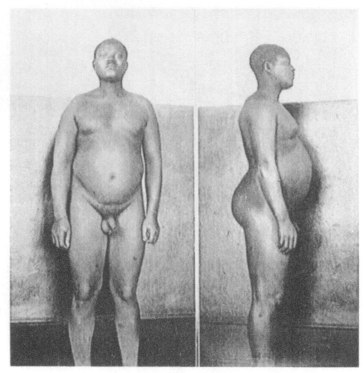

FIG. 48. Bantu-Pyknic.

dysplastics. This we did because they seem to differ somatically and mentally from the tall, well-proportioned athletics, and to correspond in these respects to the dysplastics. The stout, muscular athletics we have not treated intensively. This is not because they are unimportant in delinquency. On the contrary, they seem to be inclined to premature and hyper-sexuality, and in some cases to situation-querulancy. But the approach was difficult, because in many cases we took them for athletic-pyknic mixtures. In juveniles where the fat, beard, etc., are not yet developed, it is extremely difficult to distinguish between this muscular thick-set group and the well-trained muscular pyknics. Kretschmer does not describe them separately. He only mentions the plump pasty athletics, ill-proportioned and with a diffuse development of fat which obscures the muscle relief.[1] The thick-set muscular group undoubtedly has some affinities with pyknics. Somatically they differ from juvenile pyknics mainly in muscularity, particularly as regards the trapezius muscles. It is a group which must be further investigated, particularly with regard to their connection with muscular pyknics, and the group of dysplastics described above. According to our observations their essential mental qualities are the following : strong, uncomplicated sex-impulse ; lack of inhibition; high self-feelings; frequent, quickly-passing-over reactions of anger and disrespect. Most of these qualities may also be interpreted on the basis of athletic-pyknic mixtures (vide cases 38, 39, 41, 42).

The following case of a dysplastic, plump, muscular boy will illustrate the main points mentioned above in connection with the plump musculars : he has many athletic features in his physique (trapezius, broad shoulders, steep back of skull, height of chin, etc.), but he has many qualities foreign to his type (total height, length of legs, fat plumpness, straight profile, etc.). In fact the short legs as compared with the trunk, straight profile, fairly round face, etc. seem to indicate the pyknic. On

[1] *Physique and Character*, p. 25.

the mental side we see first of all that he is an out-standing problem for society, and should therefore be studied and explained bio-typologically. Moreover, some of his mental characteristics may be explained on the basis of a mixture between athletic and pyknic, e.g. free, self-assertive social behaviour, aim-definite sex impulse. Accordingly we are at a loss what to do with him from a bio-typological point of view.

Case 58a.—Age 15½ years. At age of 12 beyond control at home ; refuses to go to school ; stays out late at night ; a power for evil with other boys ; stole a bicycle, and at home everything must be locked away for him ; corporal punishment has no effect; no self-respect, according to teachers ; cheeky. Accordingly committed to industrial school. But could not be controlled; put veld on fire ; from thirteenth year a hyper sexuality ; night visits to kaffir huts for this purpose ; promiscuous misbehaviour with every girl within reach ; sexual maniac. In reformatory : a bull-type ; stolid replies ; self-confident ; no scruples or inhibitions ; easily flattered ; lazy at work and pulls an ergogram (Fig. 30, c) which indicates slackness, though impulsiveness of energy ; unreflective. Institution offences : Disobedience and negligence, laziness, persistent smoking and large quantities of tobacco frequently found in his possession ; frequent theft of food, malicious injury to property, frequent disrespect and gross misconduct.

Somatically : plump muscular (vide Fig. 47), fair fat layer over whole body, weight 65 Kg., broad shoulders (40 cms.), short [1] legs (80·5 troch.), and total body (161 cms.), high head and coarse hair ; very asymetrical, skew body (see Fig. 47).

44. Infantile, fat dysplasia

Here we want to describe some examples of a peculiar type of which we have found about 6 per cent in our material. They are so much alike in physique and mental make-up that we certainly have to do here with a very regular somatic-temperamental correlation :—

Case 60.—Age 20 years. Played truant from school, ran away from home ; late hours in bad company ; quick

[1] It is possible that all these plump musculars are athletics, whose length of legs, etc., has been prematurely inhibited by hyper or premature sexuality (Breitmann, Berman). The same principle of growth of legs, however, is found in pyknics and in women.

tempered, threatened his mother on several occasions, fights with children of neighbourhood ; filthy language and habits. On account of this committed to industrial school. Absconded several times, on last occasion house-breaking and theft. In reformatory : fair progress in carpentry. My finding : outspoken ; boyish arrogance ; prefers not to tell me about his previous life, because I may be something other than a student ; is not prepared to let his photo be taken because unnecessary ; self-assertive ; " rechthaberisch " ; querulant ; sometimes delights in bullying other boys ; loud and pleasant ; bold ; infantile lack of tenacity and seriousness ; quick-tempered ; does not believe in any religion. In letters : " I am " style ; his return home must be kept a secret, because he wants to surprise the fellows . Physique : short, pasty, and thickset, with heavy fat layer on buttocks ; at age of 20 no beard and very weak armpit-hair, soft head hair (vide Fig. 46).

Case 61.—Age 17 years. Very wayward boy, plays truant from school ; defiant towards step-mother whom he addresses by her Christian name. At industrial school stole motor-cycle and absconded. In reformatory : fond of a big meal ; of a fighting disposition ; defiant and bad-tempered ; in school he has a very bad reputation, but makes very good progress in plumbing. My finding : in beginning unwilling to be tested, defiant, and frankly stated that these tests are non-sensical ; with tactful handling became much more tractable, but always remained a case of extreme querulatoric self-feelings ; openly mocks at religion ; likes to be taken notice of ; very little sympathetic feelings. Physique : short, pasty, and thickset, very weak secondary hair, heavy fat accumulation on buttocks, the same type as the foregoing.

These cases undoubtedly have many affinities with the querulant variety of hypomanics. Even on the physique side they have pyknic qualities : straight profile-line, roundish face, soft head-hair, fine textured skin, neck placed low between shoulders, etc. But the weak secondary hair is a striking exception.

As far as these various dysplastic groups are concerned, we only give some tentative somatical-temperamental correlations. Our main aim is to indicate the following : (*a*) The heterogeneity of the dysplastics. (*b*) Their extreme importance for delinquency. (*c*) The great scope for working out special types in this group.

CHAPTER VIII

CO-ORDINATIONS WITH SOME OTHER TYPOLOGICAL STUDIES

45. *General*

From the commencement we have emphasized that the various biotypologies should be brought under the same formulæ and should supplement one another. The typology of Kretschmer extended by the studies of Pfahler and others, must be co-ordinated primarily with the typology of the Jaensch school, the typology of Heymans and Wiersma, the types of Jung and the endocrine personalities of Berman. All these types are biotypes (i.e. based on biological, physiological or clinical principles of division), or if not biotypes originally, as e.g. the types of Heymans and Wiersma, they have been biotypologically co-ordinated afterwards. We cannot co-ordinate our " Triangle of Temperaments " with all these studies in detail. In previous chapters we have repeatedly referred to the Jaensch typology because we have really been materially aided in our analyses by their accurate studies, and we feel assured that the two typologies almost coincide. It is therefore incumbent upon us to show the correspondence in more detail. We have often referred to Pfahler's extensions of Kretschmer's typological theory, especially with regard to the principle of " perseveration ", because our school has in the past laid strong emphasis on volitional attitudes (Einstellung, intentions),[1] which, we think, correspond to Pfahler's " perseveration ". In the following pages we shall elaborate this statement. With regard to " perseveration " Wiersma has reached exactly the opposite conclusion to that of Kretschmer, Pfahler, ourselves and others. We must therefore

---

[1] Störring, *Psychologie* ; Skawran, *Furcht und Angst* ; *Typologie der Ergogramme.*

discuss the value of this as well as some other results reached by Wiersma on the basis of his "enquêtes". In this connection we shall refer to Jung's typology which seems to support that of Kretschmer and to contradict Wiersma's results. In the chapter on the biophysiological basis of the "Triangle of Temperaments", we shall outline our relations with the endocrine types of Berman.

46. Relations between Jaensch and Kretschmer

W. Jaensch, though very critically inclined towards Kretschmer's method of approach, viz. by way of the higher processes (feelings, intentions, thinking, etc.), and K's "grob somatischen" and "anatomischen Habitus" and anthropometric types,[1] admits a partial correspondence ("Berührungspunkte") between the typologies. The following statements by W. Jaensch prove this [2]: "B-types . . . are also found in pyknics, as, in fact, certain traits of the B-type occasionally remind one of mental structures ascribed by Kretschmer to the pyknic and cycloid persons; especially, the coherence with the environment, and the strong emotional rapport of the B-type reminds one of the subtle, emotional resonance to the stimuli of the environment which K. has demonstrated in cycloid persons. Similarly, the fluctuating moods of the B-type remind one of the behaviour of cycloids". "The T-type is obviously inclined to show definite 'schizoide' traits in the sense of Kretschmer; moreover, the T-type seems to exclude pyknic qualities and, according to our experience, is very easily found in combination with so-called 'asthenic' and athletic physique types, e.g. in sportsmen of the athletic as well as the asthenic type—the latter being very frequent in long distance runners". "The severance (disintegration) of the T-type from the environment", "still ever a point of contact with certain qualities of K.'s

---

[1] W. Jaensch, *Grundzüge einer Physiologie und Klinik der Psychophysischen Persönlichkeit*, Berlin, 1926, pp. 290, 391, 144, 46.
[2] *Grundzüge*, 143, and 392. Also compare Ewald, *op. cit.*, p. 60.

schizothyme form ". " Nobody can escape the impression that, with regard to K.'s types, the B-type according to our description seems nearer to the cyclothyme form of K., the T-type nearer to the schizothyme form of K.". Jaensch very definitely states, however, that Kretschmer's types " are no fundamental biotypes " and can by no means be considered as completely corresponding to his own types.   With Bumke he deprecates the " genial artificial " connection between schizoid and schizophrenia. Furthermore, he emphasizes that rough anatomic, somatic, and anthropometric orientations, as used by Kretschmer (structures versus functions), have long been overcome by inner medicine.

As shown by us previously, the Jaensch school at present deals just as much with the higher mental levels (emotions, intentions, images, etc.) as with the lower levels (sensations, eidetic experiences) with which they started.   In this respect they are now on a par with Kretschmer.   Jaensch has also brought his types in relation with the clinical forms of Tetany (= T-type), and Morbus Basedow (= B-type). He has admitted that the normal and disease forms are connected by flowing transitions, and that the clinical extremes may be profitably used to discover the stigmata of the normal types.[1]   Finally, he has indicated the intimate relations between the B-type and hyperthyroidism, the T-type and parathyroid deficiency.   By admitting these endocrine relations, Jaensch indirectly admitted the possible correlation between physique types and his own types, because it is generally accepted that endocrine functions and body-structure are causally related.[2]   We are therefore unable to see methodological and other fundamental formal differences between these typologies.

We shall give some quotations from writings of the Jaensch school to prove that the B-type almost coincides

---

[1] *Op. cit.*, pp. 50, 67, 148, 411, 418.

[2] Pende, Berman, Breitmann, Biedl, Schäfer, Ebbecke, etc.   The structure and anatomical proportions are just as changeable or fixed as the protrusion of the eyes and fundamentally just as much a " function " as the shining of the eyes.

with the cyclothyme of Kretschmer, and the T-type almost coincides with the schizothyme, as we have described them :—

B-type (*Integrated*).

" There is nothing stiff in his life." " His whole life is an expression of his innermost being ; his speech, movements, thinking and even his shining eyes and spirited body ". " Seelische Durchdringung aller Functionen ".[1] The motility of the B-type—not so very sure as that of the T-type, but " overflowing-bright, often only easy-graceful, or again, restless-quicksilvery, and in medium limits, rhythmic-harmoniously-rounded ", " soft flow of movement rhythms frictionlessly merging into one another ". His sport " is expression of boundless exaltation. In the man is a child who wants to play ".[2] " Active moment-attitudes " as required in a spirited salon talk, but finds it hard to reach an " active, aim-directed, intentional or volitional attitude " ; " not bound by persistent attitudes ".[3] " The motivation of his acts is very changeable, and with each new stimulus he develops a new reaction-impulse which permeates his whole ego. In this way his reactions resemble an alternating current ". Tenacity and persistence are hardly found in their sport, they excel rather in adroitness and flexibility. Their sport activity is neither purposeful, nor determined by objective aims but determined by " feelings, emotions and inner rhythm ". " He finds it very difficult to perform mechanical work under the guidance of a definite idea of aim." [4] The integrated type is opposed to abstract thinking in so far as it is separated from concrete things." " He does not love abstract logical systems." [5] " Moods labile and fluctuating." " The most prominent

[1] *Op. cit.*, pp. 292, 356 ; Weil, *Zeits. f. Psych.*, Bd. 109, p. 242.
[2] *Grundzüge*, p. 141 ; Möckelmann, *op. cit.*, p. 39.
[3] Oeser, *op. cit.*, pp. 195, 228.
[4] Möckelmann, *op. cit.*, pp. 36, 39, 40.
[5] Oeser, *op. cit.*, p. 191.

and governing feature of the B-type is the hyper-excitability of the vegetative nervous system which is very intimately connected with the emotions and moods." "Preponderating happy and jovial mood usually with depressive phases of short duration only." "Changeable moods." They are emotional personalities, but with a strong emotionally determined concentration of the attention and an intimate interweaving of feelings with the contents of perception and thinking."[1] "The cognitive activity of the Integrated type is governed by the emotionally-toned coherence between Ego and 'Umwelt'; that of the Disintegrated type by a non-emotional attitude (Stellung) towards the object." "The moods often change spontaneously with the environment. In such a mood the Integrated type builds a moment-integration, a complete harmony, with the environment; but the mood may change directly with a change of environment,[2] just as the person himself may then directly become a different one." "In the Integrated there is not the sharp distinction between the inner and external world as in the Disintegrated." "It is as if invisible ties bind me to the green object." "Very naïve, given up to the object." "When perceiving a form which appeals to my feelings, if it is a landscape, an animal, a human-being, a face, I go over it with my eyes, and this is accompanied by the same feeling as a caressing stroking."[3] "Social attitude[4]: pleasant and obliging"; "almost physical radiation of spirited contact"; "open, cheerful face"; "freudiger naiver Mitteilungsdrang und grösste Offenherzigkeit," "frank and sociable," "diverse interests, richness of ideas and quickly befriended with everybody," "noted for their 'esprit' in salon talk."

All these characterizations unmistakably apply also

[1] Oeser, pp. 191, 147; Weil, op. cit., p. 242; W. Jaensch, Grundzüge, pp. 147, 165, 264, 323.
[2] Weil, Zeits. f. Psych., Bd. 110, p. 56; Bd. 109, p. 261; Oeser, op. cit., p. 181; Möckelmann, op. cit., p. 53; W. Jaensch, op. cit., 145.
[3] Oeser, op. cit., pp. 182, 183, 216; Möckelmann, op. cit., p. 52; Grundzüge, p. 145, 392.
[4] Op. cit., p. 144; Möckelmann, op. cit., pp. 36, 48, 51; Oeser, op. cit., p. 221.

to the average cyclothyme as described by Kretschmer and his school. The evidence in favour of an almost complete identity between the cyclothyme and the Integrated or B-type is furthermore supported by the following facts : Jaensch [1] repeatedly admits the intimate relations between the Basedowoid (from which the B-type) constitution and the Manic-depressive constitution (from which the cyclo-type ") : " The Basedow is quicksilvery, from this the frequently drawn parallel (Ziehen) between Mania and Basedow," " According to Sattler the manic-depressive insanity is the most frequent of psychoses accompanying Basedow." " The manic and psycho-erethical nature of the B-complex with its cyclic psychical phases." Also on the somatic side there are many similarities, although the antagonism of W. Jaensch against " grob somatische Structur-Typen " descriptions, makes comparisons difficult. The thick neck, shining, spirited eyes with some tendency to shallowness and even protusion bulborum, well-circulated velvety skin, youthful features, etc., so characteristic of the B-type, are, as we have described previously, just as common stigmata of the pyknic habitus.

The T-type (disintegrated).

" Expression of pensiveness and concern " ; reserved, unobliging, motionless features, with sober, cold, matt, unspirited eyes; skin frequently pale, and bad circulation, " frowning forehead " (Tetany face) ; " the facial expression is anxious, morose brooding " [2]; Motoric, " Stiffness or strictly to the point, measured precision and aim-certain movements " ; in some pathological cases motorical monotony or also clumsy, top-heavy movement co-ordination ; " angled, edged, as if abrupt interference of exact brake levers." [3] Attitude towards environment [4] : " glass wall, sometimes intensified to

[1] *Grundzüge*, pp. 323, 418, 429, 437, 446, etc.
[2] *Op. cit.*, pp. 104, 106, 105, 111.
[3] *Op. cit.*, p. 141.
[4] *Op. cit.*, pp. 126, 144, 145. Möckelmann, *op. cit.*, pp. 48, 51.

an icy inaccessibility, in pathological conditions to complete
apathy, dullness and non-emotionality, in normals sometimes manifested as offending coldness, in general
normality as a lack of personal-human contact (official
attitude) "opens his heart to a few only"; "Separated
from environment" (Integrationswiderstand[1] = Autism
more or less); "not open and frank, but tendency to
preserve distance, to solitude." "Reserve may be due
to real emptiness or to a supersensitivity, already painful
in his body, which impels subject to erect walls between
himself and environment"; "such a sober-plain, affectless
man may show a mimosa-like sensitivity." The mood
of the T-type is uniform and generally rather depressed.[2]
Judgments and actions not determined by feelings and
moment-attitudes, but by intentions (Vornahmeakt),
firm, "active perseveration," aim-striving, durable
organizations and attitudes; "his mind resembles a
direct current" (as compared with the alternating current
of B-type). In sports: purposeful, tenacious; cramped,
enduring tensions.[3]

W. Jaensch[4] also mentions that : There are intimate
connections between the T-basis and catatonic stupor,
and also between the T-basis and certain prepsychotic,
schizophrenic personalities. Furthermore, Jaensch
elaborates on the fact that epileptoid characteristics and
persons certainly form a subtype of the T-type.[5] This
fits in very well with recent developments in the
Kretschmer typology, which show the intimate relations
between epileptoids and schizoids both somatically and
psychically. We may still mention that on the physiological side Jaensch's theory regarding the parathyroid
deficiency and vagotony of the T-type is in harmony
with our own theory regarding the physiological basis
of the schizothyme type.

---

[1] Integration resistance was first used by H. Thomas, and is
emphasized by Oeser (*op. cit.*, p. 184).
[2] *Grundzüge*, p. 145.
[3] Möckelmann, *op. cit.*, pp. 35, 40 ; Oeser, pp. 217, 195, 228 ;
Grundzüge, pp. 162, 451, 458.
[4] *Grundzüge*, pp. 388, 127.   [5] *Op. cit.*, pp. 274, 125.

47. *Pfahler's Extension of Kretschmer's Typology—*
Perseveration
(a) *Definitions.*

Before we can discuss Pfahler's views, we must endeavour to define the terms : Temperament, character, constitution, and personality.   Such definitions are very tentative because very little agreement has been reached in this field.   As long as such functions as " perseveration ", "tension", "Einstellung", "conation", etc., have not been completely explained, it is impossible to differentiate between complex functions which involve them.   Also our definitions are by no means original; they are eclectic, and intentionally so ;   because we should first of all aim at uniformity and stability of terms even if at the expense of etymological or psychological correctness. *Temperament*, we take with Kretschmer[1] to include Affectibility (Affizierbarkeit), Tempo and Intensity of impulse (Antrieb).   The affectibility is mainly represented by the psychæsthetic proportions " sensitivity-dullness " and the diathetic proportions " exalted-depressed ".   The epileptoid proportions " Boundness-driven " have much to do with the intensity of impulse (Antrieb), and the psychæsthetic proportions. The " Antrieb " manifests in psychic tempo and psychomotility.   The temperament seems to be closely connected with the neuroglandular system and the relations of the cortex to the subcortex, whereas the intellect seems to be closely related to the cerebral cortex.

The *character* is a product of interactions between the individual impulses (instincts), temperament, and the sociological environment.[2]   The character therefore includes primarily the sociological attitudes and sentiments.   But as far as we can see, the ethical values, i.e. judgments with regard to aims, purpose, direction of striving, etc., in a normic system, are primarily concerned with character.[3]   The character, therefore, pertains primarily

---

[1] *Med. Psych.*, p. 148 ; *Physique and Character*, p. 252.
[2] *Med. Psych.*, p. 165 ; *Physique and Character*, p. 251.
[3] Muirhead, *Elements of Ethics* ; Heymans, *Einführung in die Etik.*

to the aim-aspect, purposiveness, or direction of the manifestation of social attitudes and sentiments,[1] with special reference to their ethical value.

Constitution is defined by Kretschmer as [2] : " The totality of individual qualities which depend on heredity, i.e. which have a genotypical basis." This definition is in agreement with that of Jaensch and Lubarsch.

Personality is perhaps best conceived as including the Temperament, character, intellect and certain somatic qualities of an individual. Broadly stated, the personality is the total individuality in so far as he manifests himself in all social relations.[3] Certain authors distinguish rigorously between physique and personality. This seems to be correct in so far as the anatomical or anthropometric side of the physique is concerned. But the " imposingness " or " insignificance ", etc., of the physique, together with so many aspects of motility, which are manifested through the physique, certainly fall under personality.

(b) Perseverative—Associative.

In a well-reasoned, experimentally founded work, Pfahler criticizes Kretschmer's typology as one-sided, and endeavours to supplement it. He shows that in Kretschmer's typology the " affective-volitional side is distinctly and one-sidedly emphasised ". " It is temperament differences which for Kretschmer constitute the difference between the cyclothymic and schizothymic types and which he places parallel with physique." [4] But

---

[1] McDougall and others have defined character as " a system of directed conative tendencies " or as the organization of sentiments in some hierarchical system (*Outline of Psychology*, 1926). The first definition lays too little emphasis on the feeling aspect of character and the latter perhaps neglects the conative or active side of the character. Accordingly we tried to do justice to both the conative and the affective aspects by saying attitudes (by which we mean forms of willing) and sentiments (summation centres of feelings). Störring, *Psychologie*, pp. 191, 242.

[2] *Physique and Character*, p. 251 ; Pfahler, *op. cit.*, p. 160 ; Hoffmann *Charakteraufbaues*, p. 166 ; W. Jaensch, *op. cit.*, pp. 51, 325.

[3] J. C. Smuts, *Holism and Evolution*, London, 1927, p. 274. Smuts emphasizes that for the science of "personology" various aspects of the physique are also pertinent.

[4] Dr. G. Pfahler, *System der Typenlehren*, 1929, Leipzig, pp. 161, 162.

such qualities as the "lack of rigid, consistent thinking and long-thought-out systems and schemes" of the cyclothyme cannot be explained only, and in the first place, on the basis of temperament in Kretschmer's sense. It is possible that innate forms of cognition and elaboration act determinatively on the forms of will and feelings,[1] just as much as the will and emotional life influence the mind as a whole. Pfahler's aim is therefore to complete Kretschmer's analysis on the side of the mental apparatus, i.e. of cognition, imagery and thinking specifically. What is more, he wants to "indicate the pre-eminent position of these latter factors in the constituting of innate types and developed personalities".[2] He then goes on to show that "there is neither volition, nor attention, nor pleasure and un-pleasure without sensations or images which carry them, or contain them, etc." The typical differences of cognition and elaboration in schizothymes and cyclothymes he wants to reduce to the opposites of "perseverative" and "associative" as worked out by G. E. Müller, N. Ach, Külpe and their schools. This perseveration is very similar to the Secondary Function of Gross, Heymans, and Wiersma.[3] Contents of consciousness which may be subject to this principle of perseveration are sensations, images, complexes of images, and also mental activities, attitudes, feelings and moods.[4] He seems to conceive perseveration as manifested in a form of intrenching (eingraben) of processes, in opposition to the spreading or flowing-together manifestations of the associative function. Personalities who are more subject to the "perseveration function" would therefore tend to a system of firm images, opinions, ideas, between which there are no easy connections, and to consequential thinking and a critical analysis of new experiences with

---

[1] G. Pfahler, *op. cit.*, pp.161 and 167.
[2] Pfahler, p. 191.
[3] Pfahler, pp. 197, 203 ; C. Spearman, *Abilities of Man*, 1927, p. 43 ; Heymans and Wiersma, *op. cit* ; Brugmans, *Methoden en Begrippen* ; O. Gross, *Die Zerebrale Sekundärfunction*, 1902.
[4] Pfahler, p. 201, 202.

regard to their insertion in one or other of the image complexes.[1] This corresponds to the schizo-type. Predominance of the associative function tends towards numerous connection-possibilities the evoking of a multiplicity of image-complexes by the same stimulus, continual change of ideas and experiences, a loose structure of all connected images, easy and flowing imagery processes. Such is the cyclo-type. On the basis of these fundamental differences in cognition and elaboration, as a result of " perseveration-association ",[2] Pfahler proposes a partial explanation of such characteristic differences between the types as autism, humour, pedanticism, fanaticism, cheerfulness, literary tendencies, etc. By very ingenious experiments (senseful connections between words, blot interpretations, story-making, etc.) he shows further that schizothymes are definitely more subject to " perseveration " than cyclothymes.[3]

(c) *Perseveration and Feeling-states.*

The problem is not so simple and easily solved as Pfahler's theory of intrenching (eingraben) of all mental processes would make it. Störring [4] has shown that in pathologically fixed ideas (obsessions), their fixation and their continual reappearance in consciousness are due to feeling-states connected with the ideas. The feelings fixate the cognitive processes in consciousness. Moreover, Störring has shown that feeling-states occupying a person's consciousness, not only act reproductively and fixatingly on those cognitive contents which originally produced the feeling-state or which were definitely connected with the feeling state ; but a feeling-state acts reproductively and fixatingly on all cognitive contents which are connected with a similar feeling-state as that which at the time occupies consciousness. Accordingly,

---

[1] Pfahler, *op. cit.*, pp. 204, 205, 206, 211.
[2] *Op. cit.*, p. 219.
[3] *Op. cit.*, p. 311.
[4] *Psych. des menschlichen Gefühlslebens*, Bonn, 1915 and 1922, p. 124 ; *Psychologie*, Leipzig, 1923, pp. 194, 259.

the manic's pleasure feelings and exalted mood favour the reproduction and fixation of cognitive contents which are connected with pleasure-feelings. Melancholic patients only reproduce and have fixated in consciousness, ideas and images connected with unpleasure-feelings. The manic's "flight of ideas" (i.e. easy associative transitions, multiplicity of possible associations, changeability of ideas and images in Pfahler's sense) he explains thus: The exalted mood intensifies the feelings of pleasure— in normal moods of medium intensity only—which are connected to various ideas and images. The increased number of cognitive contents connected with intense feelings of pleasure manifests as increased interests in diverse directions. All the images and ideas which— as a result of the exalted mood—are connected with intense feelings of pleasure, are now ushered into consciousness by the selective reproduction and fixation of the ruling exalted mood. Ideas and images connected with other types of feelings or moods are selectively inhibited by the ruling exalted mood. Moreover, the pleasurable state of the mind goes parallel with an increased blood supply of the brain (Störring, Mosso),[1] and therefore a greater metabolistic turnover. The result is a strong competition among the pleasurable images for a place in consciousness and a rapid change, succession, of conscious contents. In a melancholic mood there is also fixation of unpleasant ideas, but the change of ideas is less rapid owing to the lack of extroverted interests—a privilege of pleasure states—and a low blood supply with a lowered metabolism. The feelings so characteristic of cyclothymes accordingly explain some of the fundamental cognitive peculiarities of cyclothymes.

(d) *Perseveration and Volitional Attitudes.*

In Störring's psychology there is, however, another very important type of fixation and " perseveration "

---

[1] Störring, *Psychologie*, p. 193.

which we believe is very similar to what Pfahler proposes. Störring [1] shows that in all attention processes there is a will-factor. In attention processes of adult human beings the actual attentive activity is preceded by some form of intention or act of will to attend. Such an intention may be defined " as an idea of some future activity by the subject " with which idea is connected feelings, sensations of tension and excitement. These feelings, etc., urge (impel, drive) towards the realization of the aim or future activity. In the attention process of adults we find that the actual attentive activity (i.e. thinking, scrutinizing, etc.) is preceded by some form of an idea or presentation of a future mental occupation with some object. During the process of attentive activity this idea of aim, idea of a future mental activity, recedes into the background of consciousness and from there acts determiningly or constellatively on the contents of focal consciousness. The " intention " when it has receded into the background ("Sphäre" of Kretschmer [2] and Schilder) of consciousness, from where it functions determiningly, is called a " volitional attitude " or Einstellung by Störring, Skawran, and their school. Such attitudes are of primary importance for studies in personality. Old-standing attitudes influence new ideas of aim and accordingly acts of will. Our whole life is really a constant interplay, releasing and establishing of " intentions " which recede into the background and from there act as attitudes. All the " perseveration functions" of Pfahler can be reduced to the functions of intentions or attitudes. He indicates in various places [3] the functional significance of " directing motive ", perseveration "eines Leitgedankens", perseverating image-constellation ; " innere Einstellung (Aufgabe, Instruktion, Absicht, usw.)," " perseveration of instruction." The

[1] *Psychologie*, p. 242 ; Skawran, *Experimentelle Untersuchungen über den Willen* ; *Furcht und Angst in frühen Kindesalter* ; *Typology of Ergograms*.

[2] *Med. Psychologie*, p. 97.

[3] Pfahler, *op. cit.*, pp. 246, 245, 275, 279, 308, 285, 244, etc. The "Einstellung" of Störring is identical to Lewin's Quasibedurfnis (*Vorsatz, Wille und Bedurfnis*, Berlin, 1926).

schizothyme when presented with a task, forms an "intention" or "volitional attitude" and this structure has a strong functional influence on the succeeding contents of consciousness in so far as these contents are relevant to the attitude. In cyclothymes, however, intentions are relatively insignificant as compared with the following other functions : Emotional connections between contents of consciousness as explained above ; emotional fixations without strong dynamic moment ; emotional integration with the environment (passive attitude) ; simple association. These conditions in the schizo- and cyclothymes have been very well studied on the corresponding types of Jaensch and his school. In tachistoscopic interpretation experiments Oeser has clearly shown the following [1] : The Integrated (= cyclo-) type has a naïve, given-up-to-the-object tendency, is influenced by feelings, moods, immediate environment and overflowing associations (passive attitude). The Disintegrated (= schizo-) type on the other hand is determined by active attitudes which are based on "an act of intention" (Vornahmeakt). Both types behave according to attitudes in Oeser's wider sense of the term. But the one is more a passive, receptive, intentionless, emotional, naïve self-feeling attitude ; an attitude whose intrinsic aim is harmony between the whole subject and the whole object (psychophysical integration). The other is a volitional attitude, a functioning intention, an aim-directed tension-state. In Oeser's experiments it also became manifest that images may perseverate in the cyclotype. This perseveration, however, was not willed or intended, but, with regard to the ego, was a passive perseveration. In fact, this type had great difficulty in counteracting this passive perseveration of images by an intentional corrective attitude.[2] But also with regard to the types of Kretschmer, Enke too has emphasized perseveration of "intentions".[3]

[1] Oeser, *op. cit.*, pp. 216, 161, 229.   Vide also, E. R. Jaensch, in "Feelings and Emotions," *Wittenberg Symposium*, Clark Univ., 1928.
[2] Oeser, *op. cit.*, p. 161.
[3] Enke, *op. cit.*, pp. 248, 254, also Kretschmer, *Med. Psych.*, p. 158.

(e) Skawran's Fundamental Attitude.

It may be contended that if "intentions" characterize all acts of attention, and if cyclothymes are characterized by a lack of "intentions" in our sense, the attention process of cyclothymes remains inexplicable. Without an extension of Störring's theory in this respect, this problem and also the problem of attention processes in children and animals would be unsolved. Skawran,[1] however, has lately solved this. On the basis of studies of children he has shown that there is another attitude responsible for attention processes, curiosity—under certain circumstances—fear, play, etc. This mechanism he calls "The fundamental attitude to apperceive (cognize) changes, environmental and internal organic, and to adapt to them". The first aim of this instinctive or innate attitude is harmonious relations between the organism and the environment, both on the physical and mental planes (psychophysical equilibrium or psychophysical integration). In the young child, the fundamental attitude is very pronounced. Failure to adequately apperceive or cognize a change is manifested in some or all of the following phases of preliminary adaptation : Fear (flight) ; curiosity (scrutiny) ; play and experimentation ; etc.[2] Adequate apperception or cognition is followed by more specialized adaptations according to the sex-, foodseeking-, fear-, anger-, gregarious-, or other impulses evoked. In the course of development—as Ach and Pfahler admit with regard to the perseveration of intentions [3]—intentional attitudes (Skawran : general and special attitudes) develop as a result of formal and special intentions (acts of will). These volitional attitudes become more and more complex. It is fairly obvious that the naïve, easy, given-up-to-the-environment qualities of the

[1] Skawran, *Furcht und Angst im frühen Kindesalter*, 1930.
[2] Skawran claims to have found that there are differences in reaction or preliminary adaptation between leptosomic and pyknic infants ; Leptosomes show more careful, timid curiosity, Pyknics react more with self-confident enjoying, play, or experimentation.
[3] Pfahler, *op. cit.*, p. 201. Vide also Lewin, *Vorsatz, Wille und Bedurfnis.*

cyclothyme has much in it of this " fundamental attitude " to establish psycho-organic equilibrium with the environment.   But a certain proof of the cyclothyme's extreme tendency to apperceive and impulsively (instinctively, emotionally, without intentional determinants) adapt to each new situation (external or internal) is given by the investigations of the Jaensch school : The following characterizations indicate definitely that the B-type (cyclothyme) is more subject to the fundamental innate attitude found by Skawran in early childhood, and the T-type (schizothymes) more subject to general and special intentional attitudes.[1]   " The T-type is characterized by aim-striving and high grade attention-tensions, the B-type by reflex-like reactions in which consciousness takes a passive attitude," " Striving towards a coherence between inner and external world," in the B-type, " the typical tendency to bring all the objectively given into a senseful configuration with the momentary personality-cross-section."   The psycho-physical integration, or tendency (striving, natural impulse, inclination) of the B-type to psychophysical harmony, is more or less identical to Skawran's " fundamental attitude to apperceive (cognize) and adapt to changes ".   This attitude, so strongly functioning in cyclothymes, makes them susceptible to distractions as van der Horst has shown.[2]   As. W. Jaensch repeatedly shows, the vegetative susceptibility (i.e. emotionality) of the B-type is intimately connected with the tendency to psychophysical integration.   In fact, vegetative susceptibility, emotional (instinctive) adaptation, naïve fusion of external and inner world, are only different aspects of the same fundamental biological complex.   This biological complex is also present in the schizo-group, but, relative to " intentional attitudes ", in a much less pronounced degree.   Similarly, intentional attitudes also have their indispensable functions in the mind of the cyclothyme: No thinking is possible without

---

[1] Oeser, *op. cit.* ; Weil, *op. cit.* ; Möckelmann, *op. cit.* ; W. Jaensch, *Grundzüge.*
[2] L. van der Horst, *Zt. f. Neur und Psych.*, Bd. 93, p.356.

an intentional attitude.[1] It is only a matter of " relative dominance ". Jaensch and Kretschmer also emphasize this relative dominance with regard to their divisions.

We have analysed a volitional attitude as an act of will, an intention, receded to the background of consciousness whence it acts determiningly on relevant processes of consciousness. The perseverating complex is therefore not only images of aims, but connected with them are feelings, tensions and excitement. According to Störring's analysis, these latter processes are the real fixating agents. The relative permanency, functional persistence, " perseveration " of these volitional attitudes in the schizo-type may be due to the relative weakness of feelings and emotions (vegetative stigmatization) in the schizos as compared with the cyclos, and the relative predominance of tension and excitement in the schizos. But, as we shall see in the following chapter, it is possible that all these qualities are etiologically connected with a fundamental difference in the neural and endocrine make-up of these types.

(f) Conclusions.

Our conclusions are accordingly :—

(a) It is dangerous to speak of " perseveration " simply as such, because in the schizothyme the real structure which perseverates seems to be intentional (special and general) attitudes.

(b) Images, sensations, and feeling-states may possibly have more " perseverative " tendency in the cyclothymes than in the schizothymes.

(c) Such intentional (special and general) attitudes are not purely cognitive but always include a dynamic factor in the form of feelings, tensions and excitement. According to facts given by Störring, these affective factors are the real fixative agents.

---

[1] Störring, *Psychologie*, p. 266. Thinking in animals, such as in the experiments of Köhler (*The Mentality of Apes*, London) is also done with some form of " task-awareness ". In animals and young children, the task-awareness probably remains on the perceptual level, i.e. depends on perceptions of concrete objects and not on images or ideas (cf. Stout, *Manual of Psychology*).

SOME TYPOLOGICAL STUDIES   239

(d) Emotions and the corresponding vegetative susceptibility
have much to do with the flowing " association ", and naïve
tendency to integration with the environment, as manifested
in cyclothymes.
(e) This disposition of cyclothymes seems to be due to a
relative dominance of Skawran's fundamental attitude.
Schizothymes are more subject to volitional (special and general)
attitudes of a long persistence.

48. *Wiersma's Investigations on Emotionality and Secondary
Function*

The term " emotionality " is a very general one which
should mean the degree of susceptibility to feelings and
emotions, i.e. organic sensations and their feeling-tones
of pleasure and unpleasure (Störring).   The degree of
susceptibility to feelings and emotions is generally gauged
from the intermingling of feelings, etc., with cognitive
processes.[1]   Wiersma defines emotionality as the smaller
or greater excitability or affectibility (Ansprechbarkeit).[2]
This definition is fairly unsatisfactory because we found
the leptosome to be excitable and the pyknic emotional,
so that both could (and actually do) fall under Wiersma's
" emotional ".
Secondary Function is a term derived from Gross's
hypothesis of Cerebral Secondary Function,[3] i.e. the after-
effect or residual action of a nerve process.   Wiersma [4]
explains Secondary Function as follows : " Every content
of consciousness influences other contents which are
thereby strengthened or weakened in their action.   Images,
will processes, emotions, etc., are thereby evoked or
weakened.   But, even when that content has sunk beneath
the threshold of consciousness, it still influences the
actions, thinking and Feelings.   The action during its

[1] E. R. Jaensch has accentuated this mingling (Einwebung) of
feelings with cognitive processes (perception, imagery, thinking) in
the B-type or Integrated type which corresponds to Kretschmer's
cyclothyme (Herman Weil, *op. cit.*, p. 242).
[2] E. D. Wiersma, *Zeit. f. Ang. Psych.*, Bd. 33, p. 145.
[3] Otto Gross, *Die Zerebrale Sekundärfunction*, 1902 ;   *Über Psychopath. Minderwertigkeiten*, Vienna, 1909.
[4] *Zt. f. Ang. Psych.*, Bd. 33, pp. 146, 149.

presence in consciousness is called its primary function, the after-effect of the content in question when it is no longer in consciousness is called its secondary function ". Wiersma and Heymans found that in some persons the primary function, in others the secondary function, predominates. This " secondary function " is probably fundamentally the same as the " perseveration " mentioned by Pfahler. The real difference between secondary function and primary function predominance also becomes clear from the following characterizations by Wiersma: Primary-functioning people more easily adapt themselves to all circumstances. They are more compromising, can mix with everybody, and are liked all round; they are more motile, impulsive, spontaneous, and hasty. The secondary-functioning show uniformity and stability in thinking and action ; they are more persistently energetic, pensive, and manifest harmony in thinking and feeling. But their adaptability is inhibited, they feel themselves more solitary, they are not at home in company, and create the impression of reserve and retreativeness. They are quiet, introverted (in sich gekehrt), and occupied with themselves. Heymans [1] gives the following qualities as typical for secondary function : "Difficult to become reconciled when estranged, persistent in affections " ; clinging to old memories, habit-type ; distant future determines actions; actions consequent to the person's fundamental principles ; not so much attracted by new impressions or friends ; not fond of change, etc. Van der Horst,[2] a pupil of Wiersma, maintains that in persons with a predominating secondary function, there is a relatively constant complex of images in the background of consciousness which influence all the mental processes and accordingly give a definite uniformity and coherence to the mental existence. S. F. prevents hasty steps, superficiality, and incon-

---

[1] *Gesam. kleinere Schriften*, vol. 3, 1927, p. 269. Vide also Heymans *Psychologie der Frauen* ; Brugman, *Psychologiese Methoden en Begrippen*.
[2] L. v. d. Horst, *Zeits. f. Neur. und Psych.*, Bd. 93, p. 356.

sequence.   Unfortunately the Groningen school does not differentiate between the after-effects of emotional, volitional, and cognitive processes.   Van der Horst speaks of the persistent sad mood in secondary-functioning individuals, as a result of a sad experience in the morning.

Wiersma [1] has made an extensive study of the correlation of emotionality and secondary function with physique types.   For this purpose he used the questionnaire or *enquête* method and received 415 completed questionnaires from physicians in Holland.   His results, from our point of view, are startling :   Pyknics were found to be non-emotional, secondary-functioning, and active.   They accordingly belong to his phlegmatic type.   Leptosomes are inactive, emotional, and just as much primary as secondary-functioning.   Athletics are non-emotional, mediumly active and primary-functioning.   The non-emotionality and secondary function of pyknics, the primary functioning of leptosomes and athletics and the emotionality of leptosomes, as found by Wiersma, are therefore diametrically opposed to all the writings of Kretschmer, Pfahler, W. Jaensch, Enke, and to our own experience. [2]

We submit that this serious discrepancy may be explained as follows :   In emotionality Wiersma does not distinguish between, on the one hand, true emotions and feelings, which may overflow in the comfortable and the hypomanic pyknics, and, on the other hand, the nervous irritability or excitability and sensitivity of the hyperæsthetic leptosomes.   Moreover, such a term as " phlegmatic " is, as Kretschmer has indicated, [3] very vague and broad.   The comfortable pyknic is phlegmatic, yet beams with naïve feelings of organic pleasure ;   the quiet melancholic type is also phlegmatic, yet is always prone to deep sadness.   The lame leptosome is phlegmatic too, in a sense, but his coldness is overt, often with tender

---

[1] *Zeit. f. Ang. Psych.*, Bd. 33, 1929, pp. 136–84.
[2] Vide, *Med. Psych.*, p. 158 ; Pfahler, *op. cit.*, pp. 205, 213 ; Enke *op. cit.* ; Kretschmer, *Physique and Character*, pp.130, 157, 165, 168, 177, 184, 212, 259, etc.
[3] *Op. cit.*, p. 178.

sensitivity in his innermost sanctuary. The most calm, cold, feelingless phlegma is found in many athletics. Purely psychological terms without very narrow definitions or biological-clinical bases are entirely useless in the study of types. That is why a pure psychological typology is both of little value in practice and open to dangerous inaccuracies.[1] Wiersma's second weak point seems to be his method: the statistical and questionnaire method. His statistics contradict one another outrageously[2]: in his correlations between racial features and mental qualities he finds that secondary function goes together with fair eyes and hair (Nordics versus Alpinics), long-headedness, long face, tallness of body, long legs, etc. He says, moreover, " The nordics show the following signs of secondary function : constancy in thinking and feeling, reserve and stiffness in society, tendency to isolate themselves, inability to mix in a crowd, less noisy motility." The primary functioning of Alpinics takes the form of impulsive, lively, expressive natures, easy movements, fondness of company, great adaptability everywhere, and lability of moods and emotions. As already indicated, his statistics show the opposite when he correlates Kretschmer's types with secondary function : here he finds secondary-functioning in the short thick-set type and more primary functioning in the leptosomes and athletics. On one and the same page (page 151) of his publication, his tables contradict not only one another, but also his conclusions : Emotionality predominates in shortheads as compared with longheads as 69, 4 : 64, 9 ; other questions relating to hastiness, excitability, etc., give shortheads 28, 8, and longheads 30, 9 (or in terms of non-emotionality 45, 9 : 42, 6 respectively). This shows that the shortheads are more emotional and the longheads more excitable. But Wiersma never sees the contradiction

---

[1] For similar reasons Kurt Schneider prefers a " systemless " typology and with Kretschmer and Klages warns against the mixing of sociological and psychological types. Sociological orientations are apt to occur even in clinical types with resulting inaccuracies (*Die Psychopathischen Persönlichkeiten*, 1928, p. 28).

[2] *Z. f. Ang. Psych.*, Bd. 33, p. 150, 151, 154, 163.

and simply says of the latter result : Also this table indicates that shortheads are more emotional than longheads. Apart from the statistics, the questionnaire method, wherein physicians, almost without any training in psychology, are entrusted with psychological analyses, seems to be slightly crude.[1]

Van der Horst [2] too, finds secondary functioning to predominate in pyknics as compared with leptosomes. In very technical experiments on the persistence of after-effects of sensations, he proves his contention. We need only mention here that it is possible that sensations " perseverate " in a positive form as " eidetic images " in certain types.[3] Moreover, one cannot conclude that if sensations " perseverate " in an individual, volitional attitudes will also perseverate.[4] We have to differentiate between Einstellungen, sensations, and feeling-states with regard to their perseveration. Van der Horst explains the mental life of melancholics on the basis of their secondary functioning, but he never attempts to explain the hypomanic in terms of secondary function. In fact, manic pyknics are a serious disturbance to his theory. Van der Horst also contradicts himself : he found that schizos or leptosomes are more calculative and logical, plan their future very systematically ; while pyknics have labile moods and do not think about the morrow, but live in the moment and the immediate environment. This— according to his own definitions—shows secondary functioning in leptosomes and primary functioning in pyknics. He also contradicts Wiersma, because he states that emotionality is a predisposition for circular psychosis, the disease of the pyknics, and that schizos will certainly fall more in the group of non-emotionals ; Wiersma, as we have already pointed out, found the opposite of this to be true.

[1] This point is strongly accentuated by Skawran, *Lectures published in form of notes*, Pretoria.
[2] *Zt. f. Neur. und Psych.*, Bd. 93, p. 356.
[3] Extensive experiments on these phenomena have been conducted by Weil (*op. cit.*) of the Jaensch school.
[4] Vide Oeser's differentiation between active and passive perseveration.

Wiersma's findings with regard to the stronger emotionality of leptosomes as compared with that of pyknics, and the stronger secondary function of pyknics as compared with that of leptosomes, are also contradicted by the writings of Jung,[1] who accepts a connection between his "introversion" and the schizo-group. This is in agreement with almost all modern psychiatrists : they take introversion to be a schizo-quality (Kretschmer, Carl Schneider, W. McDougall) and extraversion to be a circular quality.[2] But what is of importance for us is the fact that Jung indicates in great detail that the secondary-functioning type of Otto Gross corresponds more or less exactly to his own introverted type, i.e. Gross's secondary-functioning type = Jung's introverted type = Kretschmer's schizo-type. This deduction is the more important if we realize that Heymans and Wiersma took the concept of secondary function from Gross's writings and acknowledge the value of Gross's analysis of this fundamental quality.

[1] C. G. Jung, *Psychological Types*, London, 1923.
[2] Kretschmer, *op. cit.* ; C. Schneider, *op. cit.* ; W. McDougall, *Outline of Abnormal Psychology*, London, 1927.

CHAPTER IX

BIO-PHYSIOLOGICAL BASES OF THE TYPOLOGICAL DIFFERENCES

49. *Historical*

Particularly since the introduction into biology by Darwin of the concept of Evolution [1] and its immediate accessory theories, such as the onto- and philogenetic parallelism (Biogenetic Law of Häckle),[2] genetic studies and explanations have received much attention. Child and animal psychology have been strongly influenced by the genetic idea, while the wide application of the concept of instinct in general psychology is another manifestation of it.[3] But especially in psychopathology, the idea of genetic phases or successive stratifications (Schichtenbau) comes very much to the fore. The studies of Head and Rivers on successive regeneration of the protopathic and epicritic sensibility were very important starting-points.[4] How closely the idea of genetic stratifications is bound up with possibilities of successive destruction and regression to earlier mental layers, can be well judged from works as those of W. Jaensch and A. Storch.[5] Especially Storch endeavours to explain psychopathy and many psychoses as a remaining at, or even a regression to earlier genetic phases.

Following the example of W. and E. R. Jaensch, we can in our own types also find certain analogies with, or partial incorporation of earlier, functional phases. This is especially valuable, because our types are real

---

[1] H. Henning, *Psychologie der Gegenwart*, Berlin, 1926.
[2] Compare Stanley Hall's genetic studies.
[3] McDougall, Drever, Rivers, Karl Buhler, etc.
[4] W. H. R. Rivers, *Instinct and the Unconscious*, Cambridge, 1922.
[5] W. Jaensch, *Grundzüge*; A. Storch, *Der Entwicklungsgedanke in der Psychopathologie*, Berlin, 1924.

biotypes, and should therefore be reduced to definite biological radicals. But we should not only give a broad outline of their correspondence to well-known biological phases : a more definite correlation with neuroglandular functions will enlarge our possibilities of connecting up with other studies on endocrine types generally and in relation to delinquency in particular.[1]

50. Connections of the Cyclo-type with Early Childhood

(a) Temperament.

In previous chapters we have intimated some correspondences of the cyclos to early childhood. We must at the outset, state definitely that the correspondence is by no means complete. The intelligence and sex-life of cyclos are naturally on a fully adult level in so far as these aspects are not influenced by the temperament aspect of the personalities. But the following characteristics (mainly temperamental and somatic-humoral) certainly indicate some form of connection with the early childhood genetic phase : emotionality, lability of emotions ; naïve self-consciousness and self-feelings ; easy, frank sociability ; extraversion ; perceptive thinking,[2] identification (integration, absorption) with the environment ; playfulness ; euphory ; lack of long-thought-out systems ; rudimentary volitional attitudes, or lack of perseveration of intentions ; unreflectiveness ; susceptibility to distraction ; tendency to colour preference

---

[1] Such as those of Pende, Berman, Breitmann, etc.

[2] In connection with perceptive thinking (anschauliches Denken) Ch. Bühler shows that the thinking of early childhood is in very intimate relation with perception. This is not due to the child's inability to abstract or to think in logical categories—but is a typically childhood attitude. In puberty, on the other hand, there is the tendency to purely formal abstraction, theoreticism, logical schematicism, often without concrete perceptual bases. The practical, concrete, perceptual thinking of cyclothymes is emphasized by Kretschmer, Med. Psych., p. 113. We should note these facts in connection with our idea that the granular layer of the cortex (Berry, Brain and Mind, New York, 1928) is better developed in cyclothymes and the pyramidal layer in schizothymes (vide Ch. Bühler, Das Seelenleben, p. 125).

instead of form preference. The motoric of the cyclos, as we shall presently see, definitely resembles that of early childhood. The shallow (or even protruding) sparkling eyes, youthful features, colour and texture of skin, etc., resemble the child's. A remarkable correspondence between the two is also evident in the physique : relative size and shape of head, short neck, relatively long rump and short extremities,[1] fat accumulation, softness of the flat-lying head-hair and flexibility of joints.

Several investigators in constitution-typology have mentioned these correspondences. Mathes [2] definitely calls the pyknic women (his " pyknika "), a sexually well-differentiated youth-type. The Jaensch [3] school has repeatedly emphasized that psychophysical integration is a youth-form and decreases with maturation, while " invariance " or psychophysical independence increases with age. Kretschmer himself when describing cyclo-types often speaks of " childlike ", " naïve ", " natural ", etc.

51.   Cortical—subcortical   motility

F. H. Lewy on the basis of extensive investigations into the pathology of movements and muscle-tonus, has come to the conclusion that the cyclo-type of Kretschmer corresponds to hemiphlegia patients, in so far as their movements are strongly influenced and co-ordinated by striatum and thalamic centres.[4] Kretschmer, Jaensch, Enke, and Lewy show that the movements of cyclos

---

[1] Prof. K. Bühler, *Die geistige Entwicklung des Kindes*, Jena, 1930, p. 70, gives a good exposition of these proportions on the lines of Stratz.

[2] Mathes, *Handbuch der Frauenheilkunde*, Bd. 3, Halban und Seitz, Vienna.

[3] W. Jaensch, *Grundzüge*, p. 357. Jaensch also mentions several other similarities between early childhood and his B-type, e.g. frequent synæsthesias, youthful features and eyes, diffuse spreading of stimulations, psychogenic elements in infant tetany (spasmophily), etc. Vide also E. R. Jaensch, in *Feelings and Emotions*, Clarke Univ., 1928. p. 355.

[4] F. H. Lewy, *Lehre vom Tonus und der Bewegung*, Berlin, 1923, pp. 485, 510, 537.

are rounded, fluid, easy, the one waving into the other, with agonistic and antagonistic (successive induction or alternating reflexes) muscle contractions naturally and smoothly fitted into the movement continuity ; collective, pattern, or mass-movements occupying the whole muscular system (Gesammtmotorik) well regulated and harmoniously co-ordinated ; in hand-writing a spastic pressure and relaxation.[1] According to Lewy this exquisite co-ordination and regulation of part movements in a harmonious movement-system is the work of extra-pyramidal (subcortical) movement mechanisms in the Corpus Striatum.[2] He remarks that some of these characteristics can be observed in young children whose pyramidal (cortical) motor tracts are not yet in full function.[3] In hemiphlegia, where they also occur, the cortical influences have definitely been disturbed, but the corpus striatum and other subcortical centres have been left intact. In precise volitional movements, cortically controlled, the cyclos are not nearly as skilled as the leptosomes, whose collective movement co-ordinations, agonistic-antagonistic balance, again are very weak. The leptosome's movements, according to Lewy, correspond to that of paralysis agitans patients, who have an intact pyramidal (cortical) tract, but an inferior or diseased subcortex.[4] In the motoric of the cyclotype we have, therefore, a relative superiority of the subcortical, striatum functions and a relative inferiority of the cortical or pyramidal functions.[5] In this they resemble the period of early childhood, and are the reverse of the leptosomes.

---

[1] Lewy, pp. 510, 485, 521, 537, 588 ; Enke, *op. cit.* ; W. Jaensch, *Grundzüge*, p. 141 ; Kretschmer, *Med. Psych.*, p. 158 ; *Physique and Character*, p. 134. I have frequently noticed that in swimming where a complicated collective motorium (Gesammtmotorik) takes place, pure leptosomes are much less able than pyknics and young children to co-ordinate the breathing, arm, body, head, and leg movements harmoniously. Vide also Möckelmann, *op. cit.*, and Enke.

[2] Lewy, pp. 170, 400, 485, 537, 411, 510.

[3] Lewy, p. 97 ; Jaensch, p. 344.

[4] Lewy calls it " Adiadochokinese ", pp. 126, 485, 537.

[5] It is noteworthy that W. Jaensch reaches the opposite view in this respect. He makes the B-type " vegetative stigmatized " yet a cortical or cortiform type, and the T-type a subcortiform type. He notes himself that his conclusion in this respect is contradicted by

52. *Vegetative Stigmatization of Cyclotype*

The striatum which plays such an important part in the motility of cyclos, is also very· closely connected with the autonomic (vegetative) nervous system and the emotions and feelings.[1] In fact, the question has repeatedly been raised whether these parts of the subcortex are motor or vegetative organs. The vegetative components of all emotional or instinctive reactions depend on this system. " In the phylogenetically very old Striatum all unconscious instinctive reactions—both motor and autonomic—are co-ordinated," says Lewy. The regulation of blood-sugar, water-distribution in muscles, body temperature, Ca-K-ion balance, metabolism, endocrine functions, etc., depend on striatum and thalamic centres. The investigations of Cannon and Head [2] have proved definitely that the organic changes accompanying emotions and feelings are very closely connected with the striatum and thalamus. The striatum, globus pallidum and thalamus, i.e. the diencephalon and the basal ganglia, contain the highest centres of the autonomic nervous system and the extra-pyramidal (i.e. subcortical) movement co-ordinations. Cyclos show both an exquisite extra-pyramidal movement-co-ordination and vegetative stigmatization or emotionality.[3] I.e. the sub-cortical centres which co-ordinate and regulate collective (mass) movements, and which control organic changes accompanying emotions and feelings, respond promptly

Lewy. Oeser, *op. cit.*, a student of E. R. Jaensch, in very intensive experiments, however, also comes to the conclusion that the B-type acts and perceives according to a subcortical " Einstellung " while the T-type has a cortical "Einstellung ". Oeser accordingly contradicts W. Jaensch and supports our interpretation.

[1] Kuntz, *The Autonomic Nervous System*, Philadelphia, 1929, pp. 83, 440 ; Lewy, pp. 392, 401, 411, 552, etc. ; W. Jaensch, pp. 301, 363 ; Kretschmer, *Med. Psych.*, p. 56.

[2] Cannon, *Bodily Changes*, 1929 ; Kretschmer, *Med. Psych.*, p. 22. The thalamus seems to be more of a sensory or receptor station. the strio-pallidary system more of a motor or effector organ.

[3] There are very interesting correspondences between the typical woman, the cyclotype and the child : emotionality, fluid motorium, concrete thinking, naivity, sociability, colour preference ; somatically : short arms and legs, long rump, steep forehead, velvety skin, shallow eyes (cf. Ch. Bühler, Jaensch, Heymans, Mathes).

and profoundly to peripheral or central stimulation in the cyclo-type. The subcortex relative to the cortex, the vegetative system relative to the cerebro-spinal system, therefore, seem to dominate functionally in the cyclo-type. In the leptosomes, on the other hand, the subcortex and possibly also the vegetative system plays an inferior part, seems to be overgrown and physiologically inhibited by the cortex.

The dominance of the thalamo-striatum centres relative to the cortical, and of the vegetative system relative to the cerebro-spinal system seems also to be evident from experiments on ergograms. In extensive investigations on ergograms of Kretschmer's types, Skawran [1] has found that the cyclotype is inclined to get a convex form of ergogram (vide Fig. 30a), and, when strongly mixed with athletic constitutional factors, a " high rectangle " form (vide Fig. 30b). Unmixed leptosomes and athletics usually pull the triangle shape (vide Fig. 29c). The convex or rectangle shape of ergogram seems to correspond to relatively strong autonomic (emotional) components in the muscle performance (Kraftleistung) with a weak cortical component (attitudes).[2] The triangle shape of ergogram, on the other hand, seems to correspond to slight autonomic components and a relatively strong cortical component (volitional attitudes).

53. *Structure and Functioning of Vegetative Nervous System*

From these facts it is clear that a well-functioning thalamo-striatum-pallidum system, and, intimately con-

---

[1] *Typology of Ergograms*, 1930.

[2] From introspective evidence we know that persons drawing the convex curves usually experienced strong feeling processes while they were pulling. But the vegetative component is also evident from the similarity of these convex curves with those of active skeletal muscles when the sympathetic trunk is stimulated (Kuntz, *The Autonomic Nervous System*, Philadelphia, 1929, p. 360). If the sympathetic trunk is not stimulated, or if in ergograms no emotions occur, the curves tend to show more of the triangle shape.

nected with it, a hyperactive vegetative nervous system characterize both the young child and the cyclo-constitution-type. We may now investigate more closely this vegetative or automatic nervous system, which, as we found, plays such a prominent part in the make-up of the cyclotype and of early childhood. It has a characteristic structure and functioning.[1] The impulse-conduction in the vegetative system is not along definite tracts, but is a diffuse one, spreading in all directions. The neurones of this system are connected in a network form, and the individual neurones are " syncytically " connected with one another, i.e. are more or less continuous. The impulse spreads throughout the system on account of the relative absence of graded synaptic resistances. The vegetative system still shows much of the " all or none " principle of reaction as is the case with the protopathic reactions of Rivers.[2] Rivers maintained that the emotions also show something of this characteristic, they are generally massive reactions " with little graduation or discrimination according to the nature of the conditions by which they are produced ". In cyclothymes, especially, this seems to be the case. They are either very pleasant or very sad, very angry or intensely afraid. Neurones of the cerebro-spinal system are less diffusely connected : so-called " synhaptic " connections with synapses between the neurones. These synapses offer resistance to the spreading of impulses, and by their specific, graded resistance the impulses in the cerebro-spinal system are conducted along definite tracts, or according to well-demarcated, functional areas. Diffuse, wide, and easily spreading impulses, therefore, characterize the vegetative system, while definite tracts, graded synapses, conduction of impulses in relatively small fields and definite, functional patterns characterize the cerebro-spinal system.

The young child,[3] especially up to the eighth week after birth, has been observed by several investigators to

[1] W. Jaensch, *Grundzüge*, pp. 318, 338, etc.
[2] W. H. R. Rivers, *Instinct and the Unconscious*, 1922, p. 45.
[3] W. Jaensch, pp. 337, 339, 343, 347, etc.

manifest the syncytic or vegetative form of impulse-conduction in its whole nervous system, cerebro-spinal as well. Anatomically the infant's nerves correspond to those of the autonomic or vegetative system, because the axis cylinders are to a large extent unstrung and unmyelinated. This condition of the infant's nervous system manifests in the following ways : A characteristic movement-play, pronounced mutual influences between all the synchronic functions of the organism, etc. W. Jaensch calls this neural condition the "primordial structure" or "archineurium".

54.   *The cyclothyme as still near the Syncytic Phase*

W. Jaensch [1] has indicated the very remarkable correspondence between the diffuse and easy spreading of an impulse in the vegetative system and the flowing connections, easy, multifarious associations and lack of definite determinants in the succession of images and ideas of his B-type (our cyclo-type). He also mentions the correspondence between the definiteness, well-demarcated, functional tracts and areas of impulse-conduction in the cerebro-spinal system, and the systematic, logical, stiff (starr) succession of images and ideas in his T-type (our schizo-type). The contrasts, which Jaensch draws here, are almost identical to those of Pfahler [2] when the latter discusses the opposites "associative-perseverative" in connection with his experimental studies of the Kretschmer types : In the schizo-type "a system of firm images, ideas, opinions, between which there are but scanty connecting bridges ; accordingly, a rectilinear thinking with always only relatively slight possibilities of off-reproduction, a sharp testing of newcoming contents with the view to fit them into one of the idea-complexes " ;

---

[1] *Grundzüge*, pp. 330, 345, 318.   [2] Pfahler, *System der Typenlehren.*

in the cyclo-type "numerous possibilities of connection, evoking of multifarious image-complexes by one and the same stimulus, a continuous change of thoughts and experiences, a loose structure of all connected images."

If we bear these facts in mind and also consider the vegetative susceptibility of the cyclo-type, their sub-cortical movement co-ordinations, their resemblance in so many respects to early childhood, when the whole nervous system is still near the primordial vegetative structure, we can easily make the following conclusions : *The whole nervous system of the cyclo-type is functionally and in intrinsic structure relatively near the primordial vegetative or syncytic function and structure.* That is why there are such intimate functional relations (intermingling) between the cognitive and motor cortical processes of the cyclo-type and their vegetative-autonomic (emotional) system. W. Jaensch comes to more or less similar conclusions. But he accepts a close correspondence between the cortex and the sympathetic system and accordingly interprets his B-type as a cortiform instead of a subcortiform primordial function type.[1] We accept the cortex to be in function and structure on the synhaptic principle,[2] i.e. Jaensch's cerebro-spinal principle of function

---

[1] Jaensch repeatedly speaks of "a kind of primordial" function in the B-type, after he has definitely compared the B-type with the primordial vegetative form of connections. But afterwards he emphatically speaks of a psycho-vegetative ne-encephalic function type which must be sharply differentiated from the primordial form (*Grundzüge*, pp. 355, 351).

[2] It is very possible also that these structural and functional principles in the cortex differ in various layers. We know that the three main cortical cell layers, the pyramidal, or outermost, granular, or intermediate, and polimorphic, or innermost, layers, are differently constructed, mature successively and serve different functions. It may be that the granular layer, which subserves the senseful elaboration of sensations, i.e. transforming of sensations into perceptions, or fusion between sensations and memory images, is more pronounced in the cyclo-type, while the pyramidal layer which subserves the function of abstraction and systematic thinking, is more pronounced in the schizo-type. Structurally this is supported by the fact that the granular layer consists of multipolar (Golgi type II) cells such as are found in the autonomic nervous system. The pyramidal layer contains bipolar and Golgi type I cells, as they are mostly found in the cerebro-spinal system. (Vide Berry, *Brain and Mind*, New York, 1928, pp. 31,

and structure, and different from that of the vegetative system. We probably have to conceive the relations in some such way as the following : In the cyclo-type, the fundamental vegetative or syncytic nervous structure and function form a narrow functional and structural fusion with the successive synhaptic or cerebro-spinal structural and functional phase : the cerebro-spinal structural and functional phase retains, incorporates, or is intrinsically permeated by a large share of the earlier structural and functional phase in the cyclo-type. In the schizo-type, on the other hand, the primordial or vegetative functional and structural phase is more completely overgrown and physiologically inhibited by the superseding cerebro-spinal functional and structural phase.[1] Degeneration and destruction processes (as in schizophrenia), again, reduce the schizo-type to a purely primordial function. In the schizo-type there is no compromise, no fusion, between the two principles of structure and function, viz. synhaptic and syncytic; it is an "either—or" in baroque contrast. In the cyclo-type the two principles are in functional and structural compromise, co-operation, fusion, or in whatever way one wants to express it. That is why cyclos are so immune to schizophrenia.[2]

Our hypothesis, though based on numerous observations, as well as on references to an extensive literature and the

---

151 ; Kuntz, *The Autonomic Nervous System*, Philadelphia, 1929, p. 48 ; Störring, *Psychologie*, p.161). In connection with a probable superiorly functioning granular layer (perception) in the cyclothymes we should also consider that both the young child and the cyclothyme incline towards perceptual (anschaulich) concrete thinking, while the schizo-type prefers formal logical schematicism. (Vide *Med. Psych.*, p. 113 ; *Physique and Character* ; Ch. Bühler, *Das Seelenleben*, p. 125 ; K. Bühler, *Die geistige Entwicklung des Kindes*, Jena, 1930).

[1] The syncytic and the synhaptic functional and structural principles are probably identical or similar to Rivers's "protopathic" and "epicritic" sensibility. This author's expositions of the two types of nerve impulse conduction, and his application of them to normal and pathological mental conditions, may perhaps throw further light on our problem as well (W. H. R. Rivers, *Instinct and the Unconscious*, Cambridge, 1922).

[2] W. Jaensch (*Grundzüge*, pp. 382, 386) mentions that the vegetative nerves resist processes of degeneration very long. He also explains schizophrenia as a degeneration towards more primitive function-principles (vide also Storch, *op. cit.*, p. 49).

authoritative expositions of W. Jaensch, is as yet beset with difficulties. We have to find out more definitely which period of early childhood shows the clearest similarities with the cyclo-temperament.[1] The problems of adult, fully differentiated sex-life and intelligence of the normal pyknic, disturb the analogy considerably. Yet one cannot help describing the pyknic temperament in terms of childhood mind, and constantly comparing the two biological complexes.

55. *Leptosomes and Puberty*

In previous chapters we have dealt with this relation so fully that here we need only touch on some aspects. In motility, autism, timidity, sexual peculiarities, etc., etc., the leptosome definitely manifests clear resemblance to early puberty as it is described by Ch. Bühler and Ed. Spranger.[2] Such an intimate connection is also supported by many other facts and considerations which we have found in literature [3] on human psycho-biology, but which I cannot discuss here. We need only refer to some of these : schizophrenia, the disease of the leptosomes, has long been regarded as connected with puberty (dementia praecox). Puberty is the period when the hypophysis takes over the central position in the neuro-glandular directorate from the thyroid, thymus, etc.[4] In this early puberty period the flowing, rounded motility of the child breaks down and is succeeded by the unbalanced, left-handed yet cortically (pyramidally)

---

[1] Kretschmer, *Med. Psych.*, p. 48, mentions that according to Homburger there are three stages of motoric in early childhood of which the third stage, only, seems to correspond to that of the cyclo-type. This stage shows gracefulness, flowingness, and softness.

[2] Ch. Bühler, *Das Seelenleben des Jugendlichen*, Jena, 1927. Ed. Spranger, *Psych. des Jugendalters*. Vide also Brooks, *Psychology of Adolescence*, Boston, 1927.

[3] References in previous chapters.

[4] A. Storch, *Der Entwicklungsgedanke in der Psychopathologie*, p. 11 ; vide also Pende, Berman, Peritz, etc.

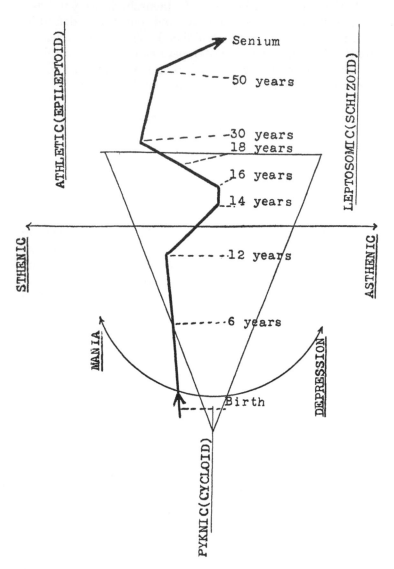

FIG. 49.—CURVE OF DEVELOPMENT OF THE PERSONALITY.

controlled motility of the pubert.[1] Jaensch mentions that in early puberty the galvanic excitability of nerves and muscles reaches a sudden high-water mark, if compared with pre- and post-puberty conditions.[2] This nervous excitability, which is such an important factor in the leptosome mind, has been observed by several investigators.[3] These fundamental similarities all point to the fact that in the normal leptosome constitution a large share of the early puberty developmental phase has been retained.

56. *Leptosomes and Senium*

There are frequent indications that leptosomes show constitutional resemblance to the male involution and senile periods. Lewy [4] mentions that the motility of paralysis agitans patients, which resembles that of the schizothyme, etc., also characterizes pathological senium. We have also observed many mental similarities between leptosomes and typical old age : the most important is the increase of excitability with old age.[5]

These similarities are important in view of the following considerations : in senium there is a de-sexualization of the constitution, i.e. a transitional stage with regard to sex, just as in early puberty. There is, furthermore, a decrease in the functions of the thyroid and parathyroid endocrine organs. This would indicate that a deficiency of these organs corresponds to the schizo-constitution. On the somatic side too, there are rough resemblances between schizo and senium.

We may view the connection in this way : the leptosomic mind and physique actually incorporate or

---

[1] Kretschmer, *Med. Psych.*, p. 48.
[2] *Grundzüge*, p. 349.
[3] Klieneberger, *Pubertät und Psychopathie*, Wiesbaden, 1914.
[4] Lewy, *op. cit.*, p. 624.
[5] Skawran, *Unpublished Lectures*.

retain a large share of the early pubertial developmental phase. They only resemble the senium phase, which is to a large extent a regression (Abbau) to the pre-manhood transitional phase.

57.   *Athletics and Adult Masculinism*

In a few instances in previous chapters we have referred to the athletic type as that of the typically adult masculinistic person. The whole relation, however, is very indefinite and unsatisfactory ; because, as far as I am aware, no scientific description of the typical, adult, masculine personality exists. I may just give a few general arguments which seem to support the relation between the athletic type and the true adult masculine form : Mathes [1] maintains that women who resemble athletics in physique are found by gynæcologists to possess abnormalities in their genital organs and functions. From the days of the Greeks up to the modern film age, the athletic proportions have been taken as the ideal male one. The endocrine organs which dominate in the athletic constitution, viz. anterior pituitary, adrenal cortex, and male interstitial cells, are accepted by all endocrinologists to be those of the typical male. [2] On the psychical side the essential characteristics of the athletic also seem to be those of the typical adult masculine personality : self-contained, non-emotional; broadly self-confident; calm temperament-matrix, which is now and again disturbed by a crisis of aggressive anger. The tensions, which appear strongly in athletics, are taken by Skawran to be the most pronounced between the ages of 25 and 40 years of the average human-being. This also points to the fact that athletics represent this period.

[1] Quoted by Th. v. d. Velde, *De Bestryding van den Echtelyken Afkeer*, Leiden, 1927, p. 256.
[2] Pende, Berman, etc.

With regard to athletics and adult masculinity we may further add that, just as in the case of pyknics, and early childhood, it is necessary to find exactly which period of manhood shows a more exact correspondence to the athletic type. On the basis of such more exact genetic correlations one may be able also to arrive at genetic sub-types. A very interesting period is, what Ch. Bühler [1] calls the " affirmative " (Bejahungs) period in contrast with the " negation " period discussed previously. The " affirmative " period stands at the beginning of manhood ($\pm$ 17–21 years) and in its self-confidence, consciousness of freedom and energy, etc., certainly corresponds to some of the main characteristics of athletics.

58. *Triangle of Temperament*

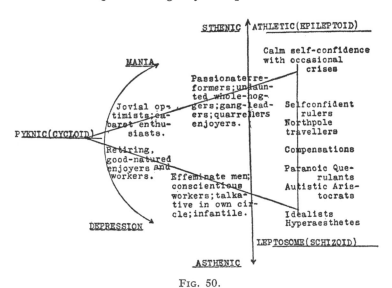

FIG. 50.

[1] *Das Seelenleben.*

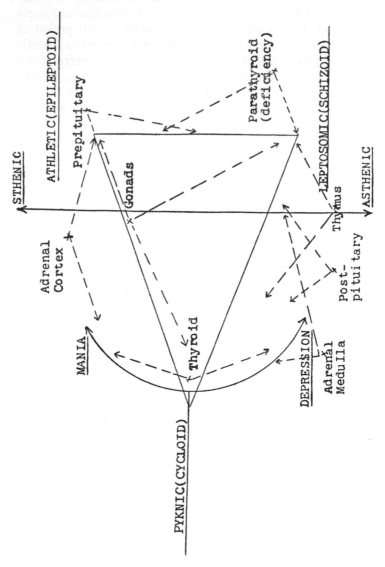

FIG. 51.

59. Co-ordination of Endocrines with Temperaments [1]

Authorities on the subject arrive more and more at the conclusion that the endocrine organs and nervous system are in reciprocal, functional relations. The nervous system and centres certainly influence the functions of glands. That is why we elaborated the possible differences in function, inner structure and biological phase-specificity of the nervous systems of the cyclo-type and schizo-type. W. Jaensch takes the extreme view that the neural differences and Ca-K-ions proportions are primary and the endocrine differences secondary. The differences in external, somatic conditions and anthropometric proportions which again depend on the endocrines are, therefore—according to Jaensch—very mediately and distantly dependent on the true fundamental biotypical differences. He makes this a strong point of criticism of Kretschmer's theory.[2] In spite of his antipathy against the endocrines, however, he definitely brings his B-type in relation to hyperthyroidism and his T-type to parathyroid deficiency. We do not think that Jaensch's view need be elaborated, since it has been definitely proved that glands as well as nervous conditions may be primary, i.e. they influence one another.[3] In fact, Pende advocates the view that they form one system. But even if the endocrines are secondary in the etiological chain, they are the manifestations of the primary differences, and from a practical symptomatic point of view, they are extremely important.

The schemes given in the previous paragraph must indicate how we have come to view the co-ordination of

[1] The works of Jaensch, Berman, Pende, etc., referred to in these pages have often been quoted previously. But we also refer in the text to the following other works : Peritz, *Einführung in die Klinik der inneren Sekretion*, Berlin, 1923 ; Ebbecke, *Psychologie und innere Sekretion*, X. *Kongress f. Expt. Psych.*, Bonn, 1927 ; Kuntz, *Autonomic Nervous System*, Philadelphia, 1929 ; Berkeley, *Endocrine Medicine*, Philadelphia, 1926.

[2] Jaensch, *Grundzüge*.

[3] Kuntz (*op. cit.*), Pende, Berkeley.

the endocrine directorate with the differences in temperament. We need only repeat the warning, frequently
uttered by endocrinologists, viz. that the functions of
glands must not be interpreted in isolation or individually.
The endocrines must always be looked upon as a constellation, an interlocking system, or, as Berman calls it "a
directorate". It is always a polyglandular activity with
sometimes one or two endocrines predominating. Also,
such factors as the Ca-K-ions proportions in the system
are important for the resultant manifestations of endocrine
activities. In our scheme the position of a gland, its
distance from or nearness to a somatic or mental quality
on the scheme indicates its importance, or otherwise, with
regard to that quality. For instance, the parathyroid
deficiency is more pronounced, and of greater significance,
in leptosomy than in athleticism, therefore it is placed
nearer to the former than to the latter in our scheme.
After these general considerations we may indicate briefly
what made us place each of the glands in these positions
of relative significance with regard to our biotypes.

Thyroid : Large, vivacious, prominent eyes, rosy cheeks,
soft well-circulated skin (Berman, Jaensch) ; labile moods,
mood psychoses, manic, flight of ideas, impulsive
(Berman, Jaensch, Ebbecke, Pende). W. Jaensch has
brought his B-type, which we showed to correspond with
K's cyclo-type, in relation to hyperthyroidism. So far
the thyroid seems to be unequivocally connected with
cyclothymy. The coincidence is, however, disturbed by
the fact that Pende takes his longitypus to be hyperthyroid sometimes ; and that Jaensch mentions the
frequent thinness of hyperthyroids. We would explain
this discrepancy as follows : the pyknic constitution does
not depend solely on the thyroid (Jaensch admits the
same possibility for his B-type). Sub-pituitary and hyper-
adrenals are probably also necessary. Moreover, thinness
with a hyperthyroid, frequently depends on a simultaneous
hyperthymus and deficient gonads—conditions very often
associated with hyperthyroidism (Peritz, Kuntz, Jaensch).

Adrenals : It seems to us that the proportions of adrenal

cortex function and adrenal medulla function are closely connected with the exaltation and depressive moods of cyclothymy. The thyroid is, of course, also implicated. Berman states that a predominant function of the medulla (adrenalin) goes with fear. This would explain the high blood-sugar [1] proportion (adrenalin mobilizes blood-sugar) usually found in affectively cramped catatonics and stuporous depressives. The adrenal cortex, on the other hand, is connected with anger, aggressiveness, self-confidence, strong muscle tonus and masculine sexuality. That is why, in our scheme, we have placed the adrenal cortex fairly near to the athletic constitution. But that this gland is not the main spindle of the athletic constitution is obvious from the fact that, the cortex type is not so tall and slender, athletics are not so hairy on the body as the cortex type, athletics are more calm and self-contained and less practical than the cortex type. The adrenal glands are certainly very intimately connected with emotions (Cannon, Berman) and the vegetative system.[2]

Pre-pituitary : The anterior pituitary is connected with migraine, epileptic brain storms and acromegaly (Berman, Peritz). The somatic characteristics of a hyperpituitary-anterior type correspond almost exactly with the athletic physique as described by Kretschmer : Large, bony frame ; strong, square protruding chin and jaws ; nose broadish and long, with bony parts pronounced ; arms and legs hairy ; thick skin, large sex organs (Peritz, Berman, Pende, Kuntz, etc.). On the mental side, too, there are many correspondences, as we have shown in previous chapters.

Parathyroid : The deficiency of this gland is connected with an insufficiency of lime (Ca) in the system and a relative excess of potassium (K). This gives rise to a galvanic hyper-excitability of the nerves and muscles—

---

[1] Teenstra, *Bloedsuikergehalte by Melancholie en Schizophrenie*, Groningen, 1929.

[2] It is noteworthy that the adrenal glands and the thyroid all of which we have brought in connection with the pyknic constitution, are also large and well functioning glands in early childhood.

a fundamental characteristic of the schizo-type and Jaensch's T-type. Parathyroid deficiency gives rise to tetany, spasmophily in children and (as Peritz says) persons who fall victims to schizophrenia are always tetanoids.[1] The typical parathyroid physique is also identical with that of Kretschmer's leptosomes and asthenics (Peritz, Berman): pale skin; drawn stiff face (tetany face); thin lips; deep-seated eyes; slender body-build; weak, atonic muscles; thin and delicate bones; asthenic thorax, and relatively long legs and arms. On the mental side, too, the most intimate relations imaginable exist between the tetany syndrome and the schizo-group (Berman, Jaensch, Peritz).

Thymus : This gland, in so far as it is connected with the status thymico-lymphaticus is certainly significant for the leptosome constitution. The status thymico-lymphaticus is the opposite of the masculinistic, adrenal cortex and male interstitial gland complex. It is very closely connected with early puberty, before it is suppressed by the cortex-interstitial complex, and in some persons it remains after puberty. The body-build associated with it is that of the asthenic leptosome. It is characterized by weak sexual endowment, frequent homosexuality, vagotony of Eppinger and Hess, introversion, shyness, timidity, femininity, easily moved to tears (Peritz, Berman). Peritz also mentions that it is closely related with the parathyroid insufficiency or tetany constitution.

Post-pituitary : This gland is also probably related to leptosomy (schizoidy), and to the more asthenic group of pyknics for the following reasons : It has to do with tender-heartedness, suggestibility, sentimentalism, feminism, sex-difficulties, according to Berman. Its hormone (pituitrin) has the same action on blood-sugar as that of the acute fear gland, adrenal medulla (adrenalin) ; only, it acts more slowly. It may therefore be related to the characterological fearsomeness and high blood-sugar of the catatonics and perhaps also of the melancholics.

---

[1] Peritz, *op. cit.*, p. 250.

The Gonads : The male interstitial glands derive from the same embryonic layer as the adrenal cortex, the muscles and the bones, viz. the mesoderm. It is natural, therefore, to find the sex glands in the male in close relationship with aggressive self-confidence, muscular people, such as the athletics and the hypo-manic pyknics. The leptosomes (or schizo-type in its purest form) being related to the status thymico-lymphaticus and tetany, certainly have the weakest and the most aim-uncertain sex-impulse. The weak or abnormal sexuality of leptosomes and the significance of interstitial gland dysfunctions in the etiology of schizoidy have been emphasized by Kretschmer, Kronfeld, and others. It is for these reasons that, in our scheme, we place hyperfunctions of the male sex glands further away from leptosomy, and nearer to the hypomanics, and the athletic constitution. It must be noted, of course, that we are dealing only with males throughout this scheme.

With the help of these co-ordinations, between various sets of typologies, e.g. endocrine, eidetic, psychopathological, genetic, etc., we shall provide our delinquency studies with a' wider basis, as well as increase the number and the reliability of methods to establish more definite psychophysical correlations.

60. *Carl Huter's Typology* [1]

Towards the close of the nineteenth century Huter had already proposed a system of bio-types which on the physical as well as on the mental side is almost identical with that of Kretschmer. Unfortunately, he retained so much of Gall's " faculty phrenology " in his doctrines, and worked with so many unscientific theories, such as helioda, energy-radiations, psychophysiognomy, etc., that he has been relegated to the group of pseudo-scientific characterologists. In fundamentals his theory amounts to the following :

[1] Carl Huter, *Illustriertes Handbuch*, Breslau, 1928 ; A. Kupfer, *Grundlagen der praktischen Menschenkenntniss*, 1928.

there are three main bio-types which depend on the relative hyper-development of each of the three primary germ-layers, or embryonic layers : the ectoderm, the mesoderm and the endoderm.

From a hyperdeveloping ectoderm we get the slim body of medium height, weak muscles and fat ; a hyper-development of those parts which derive from the ectoderm, viz. the skin, primary hair and the nervous system. This type (Huter's Empfindungstypus) corresponds to the leptosome. The second type, that of a hyperdeveloped mesoderm (Huter's Krafttypus), is characterized by such mesodermic derivations as strong muscles, heavy bones, good blood-system, dominating sex glands, etc. The third type (Huter's Ernährungstypus) shows an accentuation of the endoderm derivations, such as the vegetative organs, and corresponds to the pyknic type. As already stated, his descriptions of the temperaments and physique of these types are very near to those of Kretschmer. His theory of embryonic layers is certainly extremely stimulating, and does not seem to be improbable, though as yet not sufficiently worked out. But there are also many difficulties to be overcome if the idea of an embryonic typology is to be rigidly carried through. The great incongruencies appear with regard to the functions of neuro-glandular systems [1] ; the anterior-pituitary, so prominent in athletic constitutions, derives not from the mesoderm, from which the bones and muscles develop, but from the ectoderm. The adrenal cortex, important for both athletics and pyknics, derives from the mesoderm. The sexual glands are also very strongly functioning in the pyknic type, although they derive from the mesoderm. The vegetative nervous system itself derives entirely from the ectoderm, although it is in close functional relation with the endoderm from the beginning.[2]

---

[1] Berman, *op. cit.*; Biedl, *The Internal Secretary Organs*, London, 1913.
[2] Lewy, p. 375.